Review 1

In Ebola Virus facts and fictions, Nwakanwa Kingdom has envisioned the risk of emerging viral infections and the global insecurity.

He delivered a remarkable approach in the pursuit of a sound and more sustainable global health system. He viewed Ebola virus as a new enemy to the human race and had set forth a constructive framework for constant reminder so as to maintain a continuous preparedness against an unprecedented outbreak of a viral disease.

However, his compassion for humanity regularly yearns for a disease-free generation. He furthermore consoled those families and nations that were affected by the deadly Ebola hemorrhagic fever.

The author practically honored the bravery and sacrifice of the health workers during the epidemic.

Ambassador Ukoha Nnenna Kalu

National Executive President

All Nigerian United Nations' Students and Youth Association (ANUNSA)

Review 2

I'm delighted to have gone through the book. I found it quite intriguing and full of interesting insight about the new development scheme application in modern science and technology and leadership system.

The young man took his time and commitment in making his research. He gathered the ideal system of governance, which is produced, as sensitive information for the benefit and maintaining structure of sanity of health status in our society and Africa which is giving a voice as a ruling trend for the development of every society.

Although, "Ebola virus outbreak in West Africa" is the iconic theme of this book but the young man yet open my mind to other moribund system in leadership (tribalism, sentiments etc) which has ceased the growth of many African nation and ways to bring lasting solution to the ceaseless canker worm.

God bless you NWAKANWA KINGDOM

Oluwashindara Olanrewaju

Directorate of Arts, Entertainment and Tourism.

N.Y.C.N Lagos State Chapter

Ebola Virus

Facts and Fictions

Ebola Virus

Facts and Fictions

Related to West African Outbreak

NWAKANWA KINGDOM

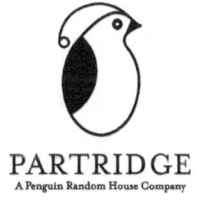

PARTRIDGE

A Penguin Random House Company

To order additional copies of this book, contact
Toll Free 0800 990 914 (South Africa)
+44 20 3014 3997 (outside South Africa)
orders.africa@partridgepublishing.com

www.partridgepublishing.com/africa

This book is dedicated to all victims of the Ebola virus outbreak, to our beloved brothers and sisters who lost their lives to malicious attack of this deadly virus. We intercede that God will accept their souls and place consolation in the hearts of their families. Special dedication goes to our late beloved sister Doctor Ameyo Adadevoh, a precious woman who sacrificed her life to save the lives of the Nigerian people. May God accept her demise and offer her peaceful life above.

Contents

Acknowledgement

First of all, I acknowledge the Almighty God for the inspiration and motivation in making this work a successful one. Special thanks go to my publishers, Partridge Africa publishing team. The support and helpful guidelines I received from them are to be forever grateful for. My heartfelt greetings to all members of Author Solutions.

To my family, my mother, Mrs Julian Akosa, and my big brother Mr Jeff Olisanedum Akosa. I thank them all for always being there for me.

My warm thanks also go to all organizations and individuals who by their numerous grants and efforts help in fighting the Ebola virus outbreak in West Africa. Special thanks to the World Health Organization, United States Centers for Disease Control and Prevention, Economic Community of West African States, African Union, European Commission, World Bank Group, World Food Programme, the United States Food and Drug Administration, the Armed Forces Health Surveillance Center, Global Emerging Infections Surveillance and Response Team, UN Mission for Ebola Emergency Response Team, the Global Partnership for Education, the West African States Ministry of Health, the Nigerian Ministry of Health, Mapp Biopharmaceutical Inc., all non-governmental organizations, Médecins Sans Frontières, the Samaritan's Purse, the Red Cross Society, the AmeriCares, the Pentagon House, Department of Homeland Security, all African health workers, MTN telecom, Airtel Africa, Svani Group, the Media Houses. I thank you all.

To all the religious people, I thank you all. We observe the significant effect of your unending prayers. May God empower you all as you continue your work of faith.

I can't forget to thank and appreciate all great science writers of our time and those of the time before us, Peter Piot, Peter W. Singer, Ray Kurzweil, Hans Moravec, Max More, I. J. Good, Nick Brostom, Richard Preston, David Quammen, Vinor Vinge, Eiman Azim (winner of 2014 Eppendorf and Science Prize for Neurobiology), whose respective contributions in science assist my research work.

To my music legend Lucky Dube, the dead hero (I call him Lucky the Prophet), I acknowledge his memories for his inspirational music.

I also say kudos to the West African government and every well-meaning citizen of West Africa for their immense contribution in combating Ebola virus outbreak in West Africa.

Foreword

This book, 'Ebola Virus—facts and fictions' is a graphic exposition of the events that surrounded the last Ebola outbreak in West Africa by a layman. It captures the characteristics of the virus as well as people's belief and attitude to the epidemic in very simple language.

It went further to describe the reaction of the people, the government and international agencies especially those that work in areas of health. It captures the mood of the whole world especially in anticipation of a world epidemic of Ebola disease. The apprehension and cooperation of all in containing the spread which was phenomenal was also well captured.

The story was laced with fictions, beliefs and propaganda by different groups advancing a number of theories surrounding population control and bioterrorism as the origin of the infection.

The book ends with some philosophical and spiritual messages.

The author is an upcoming, enthusiastic young man with great ability who needs encouragement and proper direction. The book is good for all audience but especially for the layman who needs to understand the message of Ebola and other diseases that are spread by contact as well as other bad cultural habits commonly practiced in the developing countries, so as to be able to apply preventive measures.

In fact it captured the mood of the unprepared world in the face of possible calamity.

Professor Alexander M.E Nwofor

Prof. of Surgery and Consultant Urologist

Provost, College of Health Sciences

Nnamdi Azikiwe University

Introduction

The world today is at a crucial stage; terrible things happen across the globe. The future of humanity is at risk; the recurrence of natural and man-made disasters, ranging from earthquakes, typhoons, tsunamis, cyclones, and hurricanes to wars, terrorism, and holocausts, clearly signify that the human era is approaching final stage. The effect of climate change and rapid outbreak of viral diseases are things to be concerned about.

This collective force tends to work against the fundamental desire of every human person, which includes the wish to live in a safe environment, to have access to sound public health, and to have the ability to work and make provision for essential needs required to support life. This phenomenon of living in an insecure world limits our lifespan, thereby making our life expectancy on earth very short.

This is quite contrary to the initial plan of creation, in which the Creator has made man to inhabit the earth and live in peace, to the fullest, and in abundance.

This is a cause that humans will either change or it will keep changing humanity. Most predicaments befalling mankind today are reward for man's inhumanity to man. The future of our existence is solely in our hands. Everyone must rise up and make the world a better place to live.

1 Ebola Virus Disease: A Disease in History

The world has made another history; a new enemy has visited the earth. On that helpless day in 1976, Ebola monster was discovered. Ebola had been covertly terrorizing human existence all over the world in a minimal scale until the worst outbreak hit the West African coast in 2014. People started vomiting again. Some had diarrhoea and rashes, followed by decreased functioning of the liver and kidney; others were experiencing internal and external bleeding.

The Ebola epidemic in West Africa was caused by Ebola Zaire, which is the deadliest strain among other types of Ebola virus. The first West African outbreak occurred in Guéckédou, Guinea, in March 2014.

Back in 1976, a young Zairian doctor named Ngoy Mushola travelled to a rural village in what is today the Democratic Republic of the Congo; he heard people were dying of a strange disease near the shores of the river in Zaire. They had fevers, stomach aches, and rashes. Eventually, scientists realized that a new virus was causing the disease; they named it after the river and the country. Nearly three hundred people died in that first outbreak. Then about a year later, Ebola Zaire vanished. In 1994, the virus reappeared and started hopscotching around the rainforest of Central Africa.

Biological Scientist speculate a top theory that the virus spread through bats; many signs point to bats as the main source of Ebola. The virus infects and replicates inside bats without killing or causing harm to the animals, so bats can easily spread Ebola. Bats get around; some can migrate hundreds, even thousands of miles. Although this is still a theory, scientists have found traces of the virus in individual bats, yet they still haven't been able to figure out which species are actually spreading Ebola or how long the virus has been in West Africa. Ebola outbreak does not happen often, but they are very devastating when they happen.

The Ebola virus outbreak in West Africa began in December 2013 in Guinea, but it was not detected until March 2014, after which it spread to Liberia, Sierra Leone, and Nigeria. The outbreak was caused by the Zaire Ebola virus, known simply as the Ebola virus (EBOV). It was the most severe outbreak of Ebola in terms of the number of human cases and deaths since the discovery of the virus in 1976. The number of cases from the current outbreak now outnumbers the combined cases from all known previous outbreaks. Affected countries have encountered many difficulties in their attempt to control the spread of Ebola. It is the first Ebola epidemic occurring in West Africa. As a result of this, medical institution lack knowledge and experience in dealing with a highly communicable disease. Their containment strategies are very weak; that is why the outbreak expanded, killing thousands of innocent citizens. This has triggered a catastrophe within the nations; people were expressing their anger and regrets towards the governments' limited effort in containing the outbreak.

In some areas, people have become suspicious of both the government and hospitals; some hospitals have been attacked by angry protesters who believe that the disease is a hoax or that the hospitals are responsible for the disease. The areas highly infected are areas of extreme poverty, where there is not even running water or disinfectant to help control the spread of disease. Other factors include belief in and reliance on traditional folk remedies, magical powers and cultural burial practices that predispose to physical contact with the deceased, especially death customs such as washing the body of the deceased. Some hospitals lack basic supplies and are understaffed, which has increased the likelihood of staff catching the virus themselves.

In August 2014, World Health Organization reported that 10 per cent of the dead were health-care workers. Various aid organizations and international bodies, including the Economic Community of West African States (ECOWAS), United States Centers for Disease Control and Prevention (CDC), and the European Commission, have donated funds and mobilized personnel to help counter the outbreak. Charities, including Médecins Sans Frontières, the Red Cross, and Samaritan's Purse, are also working in the area. At the end of August, the World Health Organization reported that the loss of so many health workers was making it difficult for them to provide sufficient numbers of foreign medical staff, and the African Union launched an urgent initiative to recruit more health-care workers from among its members.

Researchers believe that the first human case of the Ebola virus disease leading to the 2014 outbreak was a two-year-old boy who died on 6 December 2013 in the village of Meliandou, Guéckédou Prefecture, Guinea. His mother, three-year-old sister, and grandmother then became ill with symptoms consistent with Ebola infection and died. People infected by those victims spread the disease to other villages. The outbreak progressed to Liberia in Lofa and Nimba counties in the late March. The first outbreak in Sierra Leone was reported on 25 May in Kailahun district near the border with Guéckédou in Guinea. The outbreak in Nigeria was an imported case on 25 July. A Liberian ministry of finance official arrived at the airport in Nigeria after being exposed to the virus and died a few days later. The doctor who treated Patrick Sawyer, Ameyo Adadevoh, a descendant of Herbert Macaulay and Ajayi Crowther, also died of Ebola virus. She played a key role in curbing the spread of the virus in Nigeria by preventing the imported case.

The secret behind Ebola outbreak in Nigeria is puzzling. This is what many opinions have referred to as a deliberate plot to destroy giant of Africa. The Nigerian government and the Nigerian ministry of health delivered an irresistible effort in fighting the outbreak in Nigeria. Health officials were placed at entry points to conduct tests on people arriving in the country. Aside from the increased surveillance at the country's borders, the Nigeria government stated that they also made attempts to control the spread of disease through an improvement in tracking, providing education to avert disinformation and increase accurate information. Much efforts were delivered to scale up and strengthen all aspects of response, including contact tracking, public information and community mobilization, case management and infection prevention and control, and coordination. There is now increased disease surveillance system in a bid to monitor, control, and prevent any occurrence of the disease.

On 24 August, a British citizen, William Pooley, was medically evacuated from Sierra Leone on a Royal Air Force aeroplane from Freetown. The British health worker was the first confirmed British citizen to contract the virus in Sierra Leone. The patient was treated at the isolation unit at the Royal Free Hospital in North London. Mr Pooley, who was working in Sierra Leone as a voluntary health-care worker, was given an intensive treatment. Also, an American aid worker, Kent Brantly, became infected with Ebola while working in the Monrovia treatment centre as medical director for the aid group Samaritan's Purse. Nancy Writebol, one of Brantly's missionary co-workers, became infected at the same time. Both were flown to the United States at the beginning of August for further treatment in Atlanta's Emory University Hospital, near the headquarters of the Centers for Disease Control and Prevention.

On 21August, both Dr Brantly and Ms Writebol were discharged from Emory University Hospital, having recovered from the virus. Neither patient is considered contagious. Eric Duncan was the first Ebola case reported in United State in this outbreak. This has heightened anxiety and fear to many American citizens, deliberating on how prepared and secured the American health system is to combat such epidemic in the United States. Global Leaders and different institutions, including charity organizations, contributed effectively in controlling the outbreak. Their numerous efforts and financial grants helped in slowing down the progress of the outbreak. As of November 2015, Ebola tragedy had claimed an estimated eleven thousand lives with case count above twenty-eight thousand. According to the World Health Organization, 3,955 had been reported from Sierra Leone,

4,809 from Liberia and 2,536 from Guinea. Nigeria, Senegal, Mali and the United States of America that were previously affected had collectively a total of 33 deaths.

The challenges and difficulties in containing the outbreak were severe. Multiple locations across country borders made contact tracing hard. There was insufficient provision of medical equipment for medical personnel and disinfectants. The consequent contraction of this virus by many health-care workers caused panic among health-care providers, and most of them quitted their job. A condition of abject poverty had existed in many areas that experience larger outbreak. Poor standard of living and lack of proper sanitation in many districts posed a serious risk to containment effort.

The outbreak also has a number of negative impact on the economy of the affected countries and the rest of the world. An initial World Bank–IMF assessment for Guinea projects a full percentage point fall in GDP growth from 4.5 per cent to 3.5 per cent. The outbreak is straining the finances of the governments, with Sierra Leone using Treasury bills to fund the fight against the virus. Travel restrictions and fear of human contact have widely affected tourism and agricultural productivity. Many airlines experienced low traffic, and forecast of economic growth has reduced.

Containing Ebola virus outbreak is possible, but rebuilding Ebola-affected countries becomes the next Ebola nightmare. Until then, the entire world need to come together and pledge their support as the situation is already causing mass starvation to the poor affected countries. The Ebola virus is a monster that feeds on the love and happiness existing between humans. It sucks blood like a vampire without remorse. It has created enmity and hatred among people with lovely cultures. Ebola virus has destroyed happiness that existed among people of the present time and has ushered humanity into a new world of isolation and insecurity with one another. Ebola has displaced unity and cooperation that existed between nations.

It is painful for a woman to helplessly watch her sick toddler being forcefully taken away from her in order to prevent the spread of Ebola virus. Loved ones died in the hands of their beloved. Forced cremation of dead bodies of Ebola virus victims by the government disrespects burial cultural practices in many villages. The Ebola virus is a threat to humanity. The unexpected outbreak of such deadly virus indicates that human race is characterized with a predicament. Today the world is at war with Ebola virus; tomorrow we don't know what the next challenge may be.

Everyone must acknowledge God. Ask for forgiveness and beseech him. We shall declare a disease-free generation, a new world of love, peace, and happiness where everyone shall live together like a family.

2 Facts about Ebola Virus Outbreak

The fact about the Ebola virus outbreak must be observed by numerous factors connected to West Africa's poor health system. Before the sudden outbreak of Ebola virus, West Africa had been challenged by so many health situations resulting from inadequate health delivery and inefficient medical supply. The issues affecting health access in West African countries are plentiful. Lack of adequate funding, poor management in the medical department, insufficient supply of medical personnel, and poor organization are just a few of the countless dilemmas preventing many West African countries from attaining sustainable access to quality care.

Over the years, West Africa's medical sector has experienced a high reduction in the supply of medical personnel due to a poor standard of living. A large number of health-care workers, both in private and public sectors, no longer consider medical service a lucrative profession because of poor wages, imbalance in salary, and low funding for general maintenance. On the other hand, uncountable number of nurses and midwives are underemployed or unemployed in West Africa due to the nations' lack of the financial ability to meet modest salary demands. In connection to this troubling fact, many African health workers tend to move to larger cities and developed places in search of better salary offer, and this automatically exposes the people at the rural or underdeveloped communities to the unabated health crisis.

The complex issues in health management have left many qualified, educated, and motivated African health workers with one option of relocating to the West in search of better opportunities. This is to say that Europe and North America are reaping the rewards of West African educated health-care professionals.

It is obvious to say that many West African nations do not produce as many minimum standard of 1 physician for every 5,000 inhabitants of a geographic area as recommended by the World Health Organization. According to a 2010, report on health-care improvement, Africa nations collectively can produce a maximum of 2.3 physicians per 1,000 people; this figure is humiliating when compared to 11.0 and 33.3 of Eastern Mediterranean and Europe respectively.

Until the twenty-first century, West African government in their collective effort has failed to produce a health-care structure and management that is capable of establishing an average standard medical institution across its nations. The impact of long-time war and destruction brought by internal conflict, resulting in mass starvation and extreme poverty, has contributed to the deteriorating state of West Africa's health sector. The lack of competition and affordable health insurance options for the middle- and low-income earners posed a big challenge to West Africa's medical achievement. Meanwhile, the predictions and forecast in the African health-care improvement system has recorded a slow progress in recent times, and the estimated cost of rebuilding this sector in order to provide a sustainable and guaranteed healthy living for African people is twice the cost of provision of environmental infrastructure.

The rapid emergence of radical communicable diseases as we see in many West African nations is a result of poor living status, lack of proper sanitation, unhygienic contamination, and excessive pollution. Deadly diseases are more likely to emerge from a relatively poor or unsanitized environment. Drinking of unclean water and practising open defecation have led to the loss of millions of lives to cholera and typhoid fever. Most of these waterborne diseases aren't found in developed countries because of the sophisticated water systems that filter and chlorinate water to eliminate all disease-carrying organisms. Many other diseases still run rampant in West Africa and other developing parts of the world where there is little or no provision of amenities and life-improvement capacities brought by development in modern health science and technologies.

The Ebola virus outbreak in West Africa would have been timely contained and prevented if there were adequate health-care provision and strategic management in place over the years. Lack of efficient knowledge and unprofessionalism among public health workers catalyzed and expanded the outbreak. This issue had led to dependence on temporal foreign health assistance to deliver a standard health-care service to a poorly functioning arrangement instead of putting effort in making systematic changes that would aid the production and maintenance of a larger workforce.

Most people in the developing countries do not have access to primary education and therefore lack the fundamental knowledge of maintaining and keeping personal hygiene in order to prevent diseases and infections. Most African countries are in dire poverty and need urgent aid. Emergency response is highly encouraged in many of the African nations in order to save millions of lives dying yearly as a result of malnutrition and communicable diseases. In many rural communities, people do not have access to a square meal while others cannot afford the cost of clean water supply.

The rate of agricultural productivity has shown a massive slowdown for the past fifteen years. Meanwhile, agriculture is among the largest segments of the modern African economy. West African nations have good soil and climatic condition for agriculture, yet millions are dying of hunger. To many people, farming has become an old-timer and an uncivilized profession despite the fact that farming is the basic source of living. There is basis of economic development that do not increase the standard of living. A nation must grow beyond hunger and malnutrition before it would be seen to have economic balance. In most West African nations, 60 per cent of the people live in abject poverty and extreme hunger. Famine kills more than a deadly virus in many poor countries. In order to save lives, there is a need to launch more emergency response campaigns that cover food aid across many West Africa nations.

Girls' education is said to be the quickest way to end poverty and prevent excessive diseases in the entire world, yet little or no concern is given in girls' education. Women occupy about two-third of the world's illiterate population. Estimated 63 million girls remain out of school worldwide, and nearly half of them are in sub-Saharan Africa, says the World Bank. In many schools in rural communities, there is little or no provision of essential facilities needed for girls to be in school. Female, unlike male, are sensitive in nature; therefore, for girls to be in school, there must be provision of basic amenities, such as clean toilet, bathroom, and continuous water supply.

Does the African government actually value girls' education, and is it motivated to do something fast to improve girls' education? Most parents struggle to feed their children, so thinking about sending the kids to school seems like committing suicide. For this reason, a lot of kids grew up without experiencing primary education, let alone in feeling the pride of wearing school uniform. This in turn ruins the future of many teenage girls, thereby exposing them to countless social vices. Street hawking, child trafficking, child labour, child molestation, and teen prostitution are just few problems these children are going through for not attending school. On the other side of the world, kids born with a silver spoon attend school in air-conditioned cars and air-conditioned classrooms. When everyone acknowledges equality among all humans and understands that each person existing in this world deserves equal privileges as the other, then we are getting a solution to the numerous problems challenging human existence.

The United States and Japan have launched an initiative programme to encourage and promote girls' education worldwide. This effort is highly appreciated, and more countries are expected to join and contribute in this 'let the girls learn' initiative programme. According to Global Partnership for Education, investing in girls' education could boost agricultural output in sub-Saharan Africa by 25 per cent, and a 1 per cent increase in women with a secondary education raises a nation's annual per capita economic growth by 0.3 per cent.

How do we combat population explosion in developing countries with continued rise in the number of out-of-school girls? The dramatic increase in population rise over the past 100 years has been the conquest of diseases. It is projected that the human population will increase by 1 billion in the next decade. Population grows fastest in the world's poorest countries. Africa is the world's second largest and second most populous continent. The United Nations' recent projection predicts that West African countries, especially Nigeria, which is the continent's most populous nation, will be at the forefront of huge global population rise over the next century.

African population grew from 221 million in 1950 to 1.1 billion in 2013. Overpopulation and poverty have been the root cause of the high mortality rate and outbreak of several epidemic diseases. In order to tackle overpopulation issue in West Africa, every household must understand the consequences of overpopulation and its economic implication. Each family should be able to judge issues concerning birth-rate regulation and child-bearing policy from an unbiased standpoint. Women must not see several birth control policies set out by the government as a means to undermine their fundamental right on how many children one wishes to have; rather, parents should embrace family planning as the quickest way to achieve balance in their standard of living and to ensure a healthy lifestyle of their children in the near future. A nation that has too many people with relatively few resources to meet up with the need of its citizens is likely to suffer hunger and decline in the standard of living.

Sometimes, it is unnecessary to blame the Europeans' early colonization of Africa as the root cause of West Africa's poverty and underdevelopment. This invasion, domination, occupation, and annexation of African territory by European powers during the period of New Imperialism between 1881 and 1914 may sometimes be related to the cause of Africa's fall; the concept of slavery and its aftermath has kept Africa on the crawling stage over the years. The transportation of African slaves to America by Europeans during the sixteenth century marks the beginning of loss of human resource in the entire African empire. It is estimated that about 800,000 to 1.25 million people were taken captives as slaves between the sixteenth and nineteenth century. These were able and strong men of Africa who would have multiplied to protect and serve as a solid foundation for African development. But then, this should not be given much concern because Africa was gifted with plenty of resources that are sufficient to sustain its inhabitants if properly managed, from the revenues of oil export, mining, agriculture, and tourism. African countries should be responsible for their own economic and social development. Africans were driven by their passionate desire for independence. The quest for independence grew stronger and unstoppable, and by mid-nineteenth century, most of the continent got their independence. Advocating freedom means that we are matured and capable of self-government and so shall be responsible for our success or failure in the long run.

The issue with Africa's progress is back home. African nations have a lot of work to do internally. Civil wars, coups d'état, and ethnic conflicts from the newly emerged countries add to some horrible genocide, along with famine and out-of-control diseases (HIV/AIDS). African nations are not united. Strong tribalism and religious discrimination still exist in some part of African countries. The effects of having over two thousand languages and the presence of ethnic hatred are still dragging the continent backwards. Corruption, political injustices, untrusted administration, and selfish governance are rampant in many geopolitical regions. In some countries, the leaders do not have the ambition and will power to drive economic change. Most African leaders have the goodwill and focus to deliver quality service worthy of transformation, but old system of government and odd members of the governing body do not encourage them.

Fund mismanagement, embezzlement, money laundering, lavish spending, and ineffective planning in some sectors of African institution are a big problem. One unfaithful leader diverted fund budgeted for rural–urban community development to purchase of a private jet while another looter invested fund allocated for child education and provision of health facilities in an ultra-modern building overseas. Now tell me, where is the future of Africa?

African people must be willing to show love to one another, and they have to stop relying on foreign aid for their survival because Africa has got all it takes to survive abundantly on its own. Europeans were doing much good recently in Africa. They are showing great love through their numerous grants and charity support; African billionaires must open up and join this league. African development is for the benefit of all African people. The current situation of many West African nations is very sad. West Africa produces great people with esteemed potential, so why is the continent still not developed? How long does it take for African people to be out of pains, embrace the change, and live happily again? Africa must rise against her weakness. Africa must unite together and restore her lost glory. We must eliminate the old-fashioned system that does not support our present demand. If the fifty-four countries of Africa can integrate, operate on a single policy, govern under one decision-making body, and effectively utilize their natural resources, in just a few decades, African nations will transform to a highly automated society.

To the first-, middle-, and lower-class citizens, without spiritual satisfaction, everyone is still subjected to the same race of doom. Despite our class and living status, one thing is true, those who disbelieve and do evil are the worst of the created beings, while those who believe and do good are the best of the created beings. The future of Africa in the next one hundred years must be our collective prediction. Either we see a highly developed society of Africa or witness the emergence of a new horrible human nature, another form of human evolution ushered in by famine and poverty.

3 Ebola Virus Disease Conspiracy Theories

The rumours and media reports about Ebola outbreak in West Africa are causing panic. It is obvious that the Western media is blowing the situation of the outbreak out of proportion. Yes, Ebola outbreak in West Africa might be considered the worst outbreak in history, but there is a need to understand that Ebola virus does not kill nearly 1 per cent of the flu pandemic in the nineteenth century. The media and the social network reactions towards the outbreak cause people to be terrified. Many were confused. There is total unrest across every neighbourhood. There are a lot of fake stories associated with the outbreak. People were frustrated because they did not know what to believe any more. Some were accusing the government of inventing this virus for the purpose of wealth creation through medical intervention, while some may argued that Ebola virus was brought to Africa by Westerners to keep blacks occupied with diseases while taking their resources.

Some say that man-made Ebola took over as man-made AIDS slowed down. Internal war and mass starvation were all means to depopulate Africa. Some argue that Ebola is not a disease but witchcraft. Corpses were wrapped in a plastic bag, unseen to the public, because body parts have been removed for rituals. Some believed that organs were being stolen from the deceased to be sold on the international market. Many said that biological scientists intentionally created the virus in a laboratory in Kenema, Sierra Leone, the epicentre of the outbreak, affecting West African with the virus in order to test experimental drugs on unsuspecting victims.

Many lost their lives by drinking salt solution in an attempt to prevent Ebola virus contraction as they were instructed by their local priests. On the other hand, most people accept the theory that the sudden outbreak of Ebola virus and other epidemic infections has a proof in connection with New World Agenda to create a one-world government through medical intervention, health-care improvement, and national health insurance scheme programme.

This project will introduce microchip implant into our system. A radio-frequency identification chip that is built with high tracking capacity shall contain our personal information and link to our bank accounts. The mythology clearly states that anyone who does not have a microchip implanted in him shall not receive medical service of any type in the near future. In an attempt to save lives, the World most prominent leaders have recently taken a keen interest in the field of vaccines. They have established a special task force to oversee the administration of vaccines to children and adults throughout the world, and it is called the Global Alliance for Vaccines and Immunization (GAVI).

There is no doubt that vaccines have been used to save tens of millions of human lives and to prevent a large numbers of humans suffering from diseases such as polio and smallpox. But at the same time, it is important to note that the same medical achievement that saves lives might be misused in the hands of the evil men to cause harm. The first meeting of GAVI task force was held in Davos, Switzerland, in 2000. In this gathering, world decision-makers assembled to deliberate on the future of vaccination and strategies involved in the development of new vaccines to be sent to Third World countries.

Agenda 21 and Executive Orders

The overall principle guiding executive order action plan is to give the president certain dictatorial power to introduce and impose decrees. The reinforcement and execution of these laws shall exercise without limit in accordance with constitutional provisions of that particular nation. Executive order gives the government order to collectivize all activities of life with limitation to personal freedom. But it's unclear at what extent will such directives continue to take effect, following public reaction on the possible misuse of such power.

The signing and execution of these orders may allegedly give certain dictatorial powers to appointed bureaucrats. At any time of increased international tension, economic or financial crisis, executive order could theoretically be enacted by whichever president sitting in the office at the designated time. This executive order would give authority to the Federal Emergency Management Agency to control all communications and media and to seize all electric power fuels and minerals, public and private sectors. It would have total control of all means of transportation, including personal trucks, cars, or vehicles of any kind, and total control of highways, seaports, and waterways. They could seize all public and private health, education, and welfare facilities, as well as all airports and aircrafts, railroads, inland waterways, and storage facilities. The government could exercise overall control over all housing and finance authorities to establish forced relocation of people in designated areas to be abandoned as unsafe. The government would furthermore empower postmasters to register all men, women, and children for record-keeping and draft citizens into workforces under military supervision.

This mythology has surrounded the UN sustainability planning programme that was adopted at the UN Earth Summit more than twenty years ago. It emerged from the UN Conference on Environment and Development held in Rio de Janeiro in 1992, dedicated to addressing the most vexing environmental problems of all time. Agenda 21 is a massive programme of *action plan* for the twenty-first century, developed by the United Nations. It connects organizations that would require every resource in the world, including humans to be collectivized and controlled. This works in hand with the Commission on Global Governance. So many prominent world leaders are calling for a one-world government with the core intention to bring every activity of life under one-world decision-making body. This global neighbourhood predicates global tax, world court, and global police force. This poses great risk to individual sovereignty and freedom. An anti-human document would bring new dark ages of pain and misery yet unknown to mankind and abolish golf courses, grazing pastures, and paved roads in the name of creating a one-world government. Agenda 21 relates the impact of overpopulation on climate change and lays out what need to be done in order to achieve balance between consumption, technology, and other factors of environmental change. The core objective of Agenda 21 is sustainable development poverty eradication, health, and education. This programme calls for a collective role for everyone across all sectors.

Transhumanism, Robotic Revolution, and Artificial Intelligence

This generation is a witness to the emergence of a radical new social movement known as transhumanism, expressing continued rapid advancement of human technology and innovations in biological science. Transhumanists look to the future with far imagination beyond understanding of a normal human.

Transhumanism movement is leading to the point of singularity (an exponential increase in technological advancement so rapid that the unaided human mind is unable to grasp its implications) at the climax of human civilization, believing this event will usher in a new era of the human race in which limited mortals transcend their biological bodies and set out to conquer the universe. Transhumanism is a class of philosophies that seek to guide us towards a post-human condition. Transhumanism shares many elements of humanism, including a respect for reason and science, commitment to progress, and valuing of human (or transhuman) existence in this life. Transhumanism differs from humanism in recognizing and anticipating the radical alterations in the nature and possibilities of our lives, resulting from various sciences and technologies. In 2012, the first Global Future 2045 congress was held in Moscow. At this gathering, over fifty world-leading scientists from multiple disciplines met to develop a strategy for the future development of humankind. One of the basic aims of this congress was to construct a global network of scientists to further research on the development of cybernetic technology with the ultimate goal of transferring human's individual consciousness to an artificial carrier.

Transhumanists believe that human transformation will tackle basic challenges confronting human existence, including miseries and death. Transhumanists further point that the human species in its current form does not represent the end of our development but rather a comparatively early phase. According to Max More, this movement seeks the continuation and acceleration of the evolution of intelligent life beyond current human form and human limitations by means of science and technology guided by life-promoting principles and values. These limitations include fear, death, ageing, peril, attitude, mood, human happiness, courage, fidelity, fortitude, generosity, hopes, moderation, and perseverance.

The core theme is the desire to use technology to go beyond, to transcend the current condition of humanity, and to give human beings greater intellectual, physical, and even moral powers to enhance memory and other intellectual faculties to furthermore refine our emotional experiences and increase our subjective sense of well-being and generally to achieve a greater degree of control over our own lives.

This affirmation of human potential is a form of rebellion against God, messing with nature and tampering with our human essence or displaying punishable hubris. Human life is shaped by a balance of abilities and liabilities flowing from our given nature. We enter a world not of our own making, under conditions we did not choose, and in circumstances over which we have little control. We must accept the fact that we are entering into the realm of eugenics by trying to supplant or ignore God's providential plan for humanity.

At this point, we have clearly exceeded the limits of what is morally acceptable. However, an attempt to overcome these limitations may involve violating our deepest values. Enhancement options usually discussed among transhumanist group include radical extension of human lifespan, eradication of disease, elimination of unnecessary suffering, and augmentation of human intellectual, physical, and emotional capacities.

Space colonization and creation of super-intelligent machines may introduce the evolution of intelligent life, automatically leading to intelligence explosion. Typically, the means proposed to do this are surgery, drugs, and genetic engineering. Cautions and precautions must be taken when dealing with genetic engineering because it involves directly in alteration or provision of intelligence, strength, speed, and longevity.

Transhumanists view current human nature as a work in progress. Present humanity is not considered the endpoint of human evolution. Transhumanists hope that by responsible use of science, technology, and other rational means, we shall eventually manage to become post-humans. These are beings with vastly greater capacities than the present human beings have and reach a much greater level of personal development and maturity than current human beings do. These are beings that are much smarter, much wiser, and acquire a high level of self-discipline. We can imagine beings that are much more brilliant philosophers as we are, beings that can read books in seconds, create artworks, affectionate beings that offers love that is stronger, purer, and much more secure than any human being has yet harboured. Scientists' anticipation that this transformation will usher in an age of freedom and happiness is an illusion because happiness only comes from wisdom and wisdom evolves within limits.

Cryopreservation is taking place in a rapid form. The scientific experiment on preservation of humans and animals that cannot be sustained by contemporary medicine and available health improvement technologies with the hope that healing and resuscitation may be possible in the future. This may, in other words, be referred to as the future of the dead. The stated rationale for cryonics is that people who are considered dead by current legal or medical definitions may not be necessarily dead. According to the more stringent information-theoretic definition of death, death is as the destruction of the information within a human brain (or any cognitive structure that may constitute a person) to such an extent that recovery of the original person is theoretically impossible by any physical means. However, the concept of information-theoretic death has become the cryonicists' favourite definition of death. This theory confirms a person's death only when the information-theoretic criterion in their memories, personalities, aspirations, dreams, and hopes has been destroyed in the information-theoretic sense. That is if the structures in the brain that encode memory and personality have been so disrupted that it is no longer possible in principle to restore them to an appropriate functional state. It is proposed that cryopreserved people might someday be recovered by using highly advanced technology.

The emerging science of nanotechnology and nanomedicine will eventually lead to devices capable of extensive tissue repair and regeneration, including repair of individual cells, one molecule at a time. This future nanomedicine could theoretically recover any preserved person in which the basic brain structures encoding memory and personality remain intact. The object of cryonics is to prevent death by preserving sufficient cell structure and chemistry so that recovery of memory and personality remains possible by foreseeable technology. Cryonics proponents have argued that death based on cardiac arrest or resuscitation failure is a surely social construction used to justify terminating care of a sick patient. In this view, legal death and its aftermath is a form of euthanasia in which sick people are abandoned. Absolutely irreversible death implies the destruction of the brain to such an extent that the original information content can no longer be recovered.

Meanwhile, cryopreservation of the brain affirms the rapid improvement of neuroscience in its infancy. The act of neuropreservation outlines the techniques involved in preserving the brain of a dead person so that the person could reach future medical technology of sufficient advancement to restore health. But the question remains whether the preserved brain in its restored state will still retain full memories and personality of the cryopreserved person in his later life. It is unclear at present how much of the mind can be rescued from a preserved brain, irrespective of the preservation techniques used. But one thing for sure is that neuropreservation is very bad for public relation and considered dangerous by many cryonicists. The procedure which involves brain preservation in order to achieve an accurate neuro-patient that will retain complete personality, personal identity, and mind settings of a normal human is indeed a hectic one.

Recovering of memory and information contained in the brain of neuropreserved patient is no doubt a great task. On the other hand, revival of people that is cryopreserved by early cryonics technology may require centuries, if it is possible at all. A clear example is the preservation of Elbert Einstein's brain. Research shows that the brain of the great physicist and statistician was removed and stored within seven hours of his death and was later carved into two hundred and forty blocks, shared among different medical scientists for further research that would be published on prestigious medical journals.

Mind uploading, or mind transfer, is interconnected with brain preservation. Mind transfer has been recognized as the most efficient way to provide permanent backup to our 'mind file'. This process carefully copies and transfers mental contents, memories, personality, and consciousness from a particular brain substrate to a computational device. The computational device could then run a simulation model of the brain information processing such that it responds in essentially the same way as the original brain. This computer-based intelligence is predicted to create a human with high IQ that can think much faster than a biological human. Already, a human being is created with natural super intelligence; however, the integration of natural human intelligence with super-intelligent machine is an approach to strong *artificial intelligence.*

At this point of uncontrollable intelligence, super-intelligent machine tends to gain much freedom with balance and may become responsible for its intelligence expansion and future development. That is to say that with strong artificial intelligence, machine may possess the ability and will power to recreate and function itself. This subject has been proposed by various cryonicists and transhumanists as an alternative to death or death substitution. Transhumanists attempt to influence the individual mind to accept this idea and embrace this method of human development, citing that this is an absolute way to overcome challenges and limitations confronting our current existence in order to usher in a highly developed form of human nature.

According to futurists, large scale of society mind uploading and body enhancement might give rise to technological singularity. The central idea of transhumanism is that the destiny of our species is completely in our hands; this literally means that we are responsible for any change that may occur in our lives regardless of God's supremacy, provision, and guidance. So now that we have the technology, it is time to take responsibility for our evolution. Until now, the evolution of man has been random. But from now on, man can take responsibility for choosing what powers he can have. One idea that proponents of transhumanism recycle is as old as humanity itself. This radical change tends to limit our higher selves by the capacity of our bodies; these limitations also affect our corporeal existence.

Cloning, immortal stem cell research, genetic engineering, pre-implantation, screening and selection, seeding and weeding, neo-eugenics, and combining of human and animal genes are all activities that complement transhumanism. The risk of transhumanism alongside natural catastrophes, global warming, totalitarianism, nuclear war, terrorism, biological weapons, environmental hazards, advanced nanotechnology, superintelligent machines, general artificial intelligence, and economic crisis that is facing humanity in the twenty-first century posed a grave threat to human era.

Transhumanism is a growing movement that asserts claims and ambitions that ultimately seek to debase the position of natural man and ultimately replace him with a wholly superior counterpart. An extensive research and application in genetics, robotics, artificial intelligence, and nanotechnology creates a technologically advanced grade of 'humans' with abilities and lifespan far beyond that of the average man. According to Vernor Vinge, NASA's vision is that 'within thirty years we will have the technological means to create superhuman intelligence; shortly after the human era will be ended'. This intellectual and cultural movement supporting the use of science and technology to improve human mental and physical capacities and characteristics has been considered the 'world's most dangerous idea' by many pro-life humanist. Much effort has been pushed by pro-life family to carefully examine the global abuse of science and technology as well as to point out the dangers futuristic efforts posed to our generation. We should observe the importance of upholding sanctity of human life and the dignity of the human person.

A critical look at this ambition might look unserious to many people or perhaps appear impossible to achieve before others, but the fact is that transhumanism is taking place with a full force. Advances in genetics, cybernetics, and pharmacological enhancement as well as molecular nanotechnology have really confirmed this improvement. We know that many scientific experiments, projects, patents, and discoveries are good and helpful, but if we do not pay attention to the long-term consequences, side effects, or deontological reasons, we will definitely find ourselves lost at the point of no return. Tranhumanists, in general, aren't worried about future consequences that may occur from their unholistic human transformation invention. They believe that their future will divide *Homo sapiens* into two sub-species, the gen-rich (genetically rich) and gen-poor.

This means that enhanced post-humans see themselves as superior beings and tend to destroy or control unenhanced naturals.

Some transhumanists want to live a thousand years, believing that ageing is not inevitable. This act implies the destruction of humanity. It is far worse than abortion, terrorism, war, crime, and sectarian genocide all put together. This is simply because many of the sophisticated technology under development by trans-humanist have the capability of doing great harm. Post-human development is targeted to eliminate aging and to greatly enhance human intellectual, physical, and psychological capacities. Many transhumanists concentrate their efforts in building post-human persons at the climax of its technological advancement. These choices of life which target at post-human development yearn to reach intellectual heights as far above any current human genius; to be resistant to disease and impervious to ageing; to have unlimited youthfulness and vigour; to exercise control over their own desires, mood, and mental state; to be able to avoid weakness, depression, or being irritated about petty things; to have an increased capacity for pleasure, love, artistic appreciation, and serenity;

and to experience novel states of consciousness that current human brains cannot access.

It is now clear that humans are no longer the most important beings in the universe. All technological progress of human society is geared towards the transformation of the human species in order to introduce post-human era, a highly automated and civilized society made by smart and super-intelligent beings.

The invention of nanotechnology and its application in robotic industry will lead to robotic revolution. Robotic takeover no doubt is taking place in exponential rate. The timing is running fast; we are approaching the age of spiritual machine or nano-century, in which all human lives and human activities will be customized in a nanoscale. Despite the threat of dehumanization, it is clear that technological progress is driving our civilization, and we are getting close to the singularity as predicted by the futurists. At the climax of technological singularity, we shall witness the development of computers that is 'awake' and superhumanly intelligent. Large computer networks may rise as a superhumanly intelligent entity. Computer or human interfaces may become so intimate that users may reasonably be considered superhumanly intelligent. Also, biological science may find ways to improve human intellect in order to achieve superficial humans with greater capacities. This illustration agrees with British statistician I. J. Good, who expresses his view in the following quote:

> Let an ultra-intelligent machine be defined as a machine that can far surpass all the intellectual activities of any man however clever. Since the design of machines is one of these intellectual activities, an ultra-intelligent machine could design even better machines; there would then unquestionably be an 'intelligence explosion', and the intelligence of man would be left far behind. Thus the first ultra-intelligent machine is the last invention that man need ever make.

It's important to note that robotics technologies may have only reached some level of maturity in recent years, but they've existed in the popular imagination for generations, and in some cases, even millennia. However, most actual concern about robotic developments involves fears about job security.

The robot is gradually taking over menial labour job in our system. An estimated 70 per cent of human labour will become obsolete within three generations. This is simply because the rapid advancement we see in robotics technology clearly shows that highly capable humanoid robots with advanced vision recognition and motor coordination systems are going to take over most menial labour jobs, exposing future employment at a higher risk. This is more likely to say that we are losing jobs to computerization. When we often talk about artificial intelligence (AI) and disastrous effect of designing an ultra-intelligent machines, it sounds funny or looks like a joke to a lot of people. There you see people relax comfortably on their couch, watching TV, but the fact is that the industrial revolution is becoming reality before our eyes as the day passes by. We are already seeing this happen on a mass scale. Job automation is increasing faster as robotics companies double the rate of production of smart robots in order to displace human workers.

Jobs in transportation or logistics, manufacturing, agriculture, production labour, fire-fighting, administrative support, sales, services, and community policing will be largely affected. For instance, the invention of the automated teller machine (ATM) into the banking system has led to unemployment of uncountable number of human cashiers or bank tellers across the globe. The design of mobile phones and electronic mail application has affected jobs in the public mail post. The sophistication of artificial intelligence in later years will also affect jobs in management, science, engineering, and the arts. Computer remains far smarter than human intelligence, and it is making the human brain lazy and dull since it can perform calculation and run database processing faster and more accurately than any human brain can do.

Machines are already smarter than humans in performing more complex task. Futurists speculate that one day we may build a machine that will surpass all human intelligence, and this machine will later become much stronger to replicate itself, producing super-intelligent machines. Robots will sharply divide the economic class. Those who were displaced by the robot will become jobless and homeless while the powerful people who controls the business will take advantage of robotic world and become super-rich, leaving the gap between the poor and the rich unimaginable. The world of employment is never going to be the same again. Technology has already displaced human workers in a whole host of arenas, and this transition is only going to become more rapid in the years ahead. Humanoid robots designed with special sensors and security intelligence will be deployed in the battlefield to assist existing soldiers to track enemy combatants. As time progresses, this will transit to highly efficient robotic soldiers exercising mass killing at the war front as displayed in the *Terminator.*

The demand for labour is decreasing every day. Many big corporations have chosen robot workers over the human labourers, stating that working with robots will speed up economic growth and maximize profit-making in the entire economic marketplace. This is no doubt since robots can work faster, smarter, and tirelessly. The robot is always submitted to its employer. It is highly discipline and do not complain about certain things or file a lawsuit against its employer. Meanwhile, the cost of purchasing, hiring, and operating robots in a company is far lesser when compared to the cost of employing large number of humans, who may have many reasons for not being punctual or for not showing up to work at all. We are much closer to a digital world.

Computers and powerful machines are rapidly taking over human endeavours. Over the next century, we shall witness a world where only innovative and creative individuals who can out-think robots exist in a highly automated society with a relatively countable number of people at the zenith of technological advancement of human civilization.

Enlarged number of job losers will lead to mass riot, and this will reinforce the globalists' idea on depopulation in order to conserve energy and resources. The *think tank* group may target to eliminate unemployed people since they are considered useless eaters and add no value to the society. The only way to ensure your long-term existence in this future society is to invest in education and creative works and boost your mental skills. Innovation, disciplined self-investment, and entrepreneurship actions are necessary. Offer adequate education to your kids and guide them towards creative lifestyle.

In other words, it is clear to say that the human civilization and technological advancement are mere signs of end-time prophecy as chronicled earlier in the scripture, an evidence of great rebellion, the development of human civilization in the aftermath of the flood. It is a time marked by another rebellion first detailed in Genesis 11. Humankind sets out a construction project. They want to build a great monument that reaches to the skies. This tower will shelter both the former and later generations of humankind to avoid scattering all over the earth. They took advantage of a single language and tended to establish a one-world government. God foresaw their plan and went down to give them different languages so that they could not understand each other's speech.

God scattered the human race and confused the people with different languages. His reason for doing this was to avoid the inevitable disaster wrought by global government and a common language. This is a prophecy of things to come, a prophecy of something so disastrous to human race. God knew that if humankind is left to pursue its technological development, the human race at its sophistication would one day challenge him. The human race set out to build a monument to its own greatness, exalting mankind above God and extending its tower far into heaven with the sole intent of usurping God's glory and authority.

This arrogant human desire did not end in the construction of the Tower of Babel. It obviously continues today as we see rapid advancements in technology and soon it will result in one final attempt to usurp the glory and authority of God. 'Here is wisdom, let him that hath understanding count the number of the beast, for it is the number of men, and his number is six hundred threescore and six.' That is 666. 'And they worshiped the dragon which gave power unto the beast, and they worshiped the beast' (Revelation 13 verse to 18)

Today the scripture is being fulfilled before our very eyes; the Antichrist's seat will be occupied. The world awaits his full and final development. The Lord will destroy him by the spirit of his mouth (the Word of God). God already foresees the future of humankind when he quoted in the Holy Quran, Surah Al-Baqarah 2, verses 21 and 22.

> O Mankind, worship your Lord who has created you and those before you so that ye may ward off evil. Who hath appointed the earth a resting place for you, and the sky a canopy; and causeth water to pour down from the sky thereby producing fruits as foods for you, and do not set up rivals against Allah when ye know (better).

4 Ebola Virus Disease: A Tale of Nation's Weak Health System

The issue with West Africa's poor-functioning health-care system is connected to the other troubling factors challenging Africa's development over the years. Corruption and political injustice which have been ravaging African countries for centuries have become the major source of the continent's weakness. They play a negative impact, withholding countries' development in achieving human civilization. The sudden outbreak of Ebola across West Africa exposes the weakness of African health institutions and the achievement of the global world medical history. This scenario shows the level of the global insecurity. The global population would better find ways to protect themselves rather than to be totally dependent on the global government or the international agencies to protect them at any time of insecurity. This is what most people perceive as the West's medical tyranny and deceit, the creation of circumstances in which subject nations constantly rely on them for aid, expertise, and assistance. Such dependence is contrary to national sovereignty and endangers the freedom and security of individuals within that nation.

Tracing back the root cause of Africa's underdevelopment, it is clear to understand that Africa was deliberately exploited and underdeveloped by European colonial regimes. The combination of political power and economic exploitation of Africa by Europeans led to the poor state of African politics and economy as evident in the late twentieth century. In understanding this better, one must look at the state of Africa prior to European entry, Africa's contribution to capitalist development, the effect of colonial education, the impact of missionary activities, the collective nature of African organizations, and of course, the exploitation of African resources during the colonial era and consequent 'underdevelopment'.

Europeans went through several phases of desire in Africa. First, it was gold and the human cargo (slavery). The shipping superiority had led to the breakup of African kingdom and states in the sixteenth-seventeenth century leading to the Portuguese slave trade and decision-making role of Europeans in Africa. While dissecting the slave trade, the mission drew parallels between the rise of the European seaport towns of Bristol, Liverpool, Nantes, and Seville and the Atlantic slave trade. Colonization gave Europe a technological edge through the exploitation of African minerals important for making steel alloys, manganese, and chrome, including columbite (critical for aircraft engines).

A historical perspective is essential in order to understand why African countries have failed to take part in the international economic development we are seeing in this era of globalization. An important reason for the continent's technological underdevelopment is the geographical obstacles to communicate both internally and with the rest of the world. The Sahara has been a barrier in the north, and the Atlantic Coast had no contact with the rest world until the first Europeans arrived around 1500. The influence of the Arab world and India came mainly via the Nile Valley and the East African coast, and it had a little spillover effect in further inland, with the exception of the Niger and the Nile. The continent's rivers with their large waterfalls have not provided a navigable route to the interior, in contrast to the rivers of Europe and Asia. The problems of today's landlocked states illustrate the great importance of communication for economic and cultural development. Lack of political stability accounts for many of the development problems in post-colonial Africa, and it has deep historical roots.

The ethnic diversity of the continent is extraordinary. Linguists have identified around 900 separate language groups. Nation-building in Africa's independent states has thus been particularly difficult. National endeavours have been hampered by internal conflicts and civil wars. Until the twenty-first century, African nations continue in constant struggle to combat many challenges withholding African development. Selfish leadership and greed attached to politics have been the major cause of the 'African fall'. Africa has great nations blessed with gemstones and precious metals, yet no technological advancement. The soil is fertile, and the climate is conducive for agriculture, yet millions are dying of hunger. The land is rich in oil, yet it has poor power supply. It has lots of medicinal roots and herbs capable of curing diseases, yet there is a high mortality rate as the rate of deadly diseases increases.

Sub-Saharan Africa suffers from many challenging environmental degradations. There is a high rise in slum and urban outdoor pollution. This has proven to be the major cause of ill health in the region, resulting to high mortality rate. The slum is always associated with the substandard house, poor sanitation, overcrowding, and lack of clean water supply. Globally, an estimated 1 billion people live in slum, and Africa shares 71.8 per cent of the urban slum dwellers, and this figure is expected to double by 2030. People living in slums are exposed to a severe health crisis, such as cholera and tuberculosis.

The rate of child malnutrition in urban slum and rural areas is high, and children suffer the highest proportion of health risk present in a slum. Life expectancy for kids living in a slum is very short, and in most cases, one out of five children does not live to see their fifth birthday. Urban outdoor pollution in Africa is responsible for about 49,000 premature deaths annually.

Across Africa, 45 per cent of the urban slum residents lack access to improved sanitation in 2000, and 30–50 per cent of them lack access to clean water. This is a very big problem. West African governments are busy with the development of mega-city projects, while little or no attention is given to the people living in the slum neighbourhood. Slum harbors' hazardous and harmful substances unknown to the public, thus exposing the entire nation to range of insecurity. It is difficult to tackle environmental insecurity regardless of the dangers of slum and health risk.

Kibera is the largest urban slum in Africa with a life expectancy of 30 years compared to 62.7 years old of the world. The Kibera slum in Kenya, East Africa, represents 42 per cent of the slum neighbourhood existing in Africa. Life in Kibera is not easy. It is more like a jungle, the journey of the prey and the predators. There are little or no infrastructure and life amenities. There is no proper drainage system. Stagnant and contaminated water exposes residents to epidemic-prone infection and waterborne diseases. There is improper sanitation in Kibera, and most people lack access to proper health care. Kibera residents pay five times more than other Kenya residents living outside the slum to get water for drinking and sanitation. In most cases, people do not have money to buy water. There is high unemployment. There are few health centres without adequate facilities. There are few schools, but most people can't afford the cost of sending their kids to school. Life in Kibera is risky. About one million residents share 600 toilets, wherein a single toilet serves 1,300 people. This is a very poor hygiene.

Many people in the world may not experience the lifestyle in Kibera throughout their existence on earth. Many cannot imagine the kind of life that exists in the slum, and a lot of people may not know how it feels to be born and raised in such environment like Kibera slum. Life in Kibera is life outside the world. Violence is rampant. Kibera residents are not protected. They lack police security. The young girls were beaten, raped, and molested by bad boys, exposing teenage girls to HIV and unwanted pregnancy. The question remains if the government is actually doing something to improve the lives of people living in this zone, or are they forever abandoned to bear their burden?

Most people can refer the life in the slum as 'ghetto living'. Life in the ghetto is a jungle of the masters. The language commonly used in the ghetto is 'life as a survival of the fittest', the environment where only the strong and able-minded survives. In general, all ghetto communities shared one characteristic of harbouring smart and agile young people. Ghetto residents are not scared to face life since life has exposed them to a situation that they neither chose nor have the ability to change; hence, they strive to live beyond all odds. Slum dwellers struggle to exist in spite of all afflictions and burdens which life has placed on them.

Today, our modern ghetto has turned out to become an environment of serious people. Both children and the adults were very much serious. Everyone is ready for the next challenge of life. The condition of dire poverty has led a lot people to commit crimes and all sorts of social vices in their irresistible attempt to live. How do you feel to wake up in the morning to realize that you have less than one dollar to pay your daily bills, yet you are unemployed? What is likely to be the solution to this situation? To stay idle and die of hunger? To apply for a job without primary education, even when uncountable number of university graduates are unemployed? This situation has led many young people into frustration and crime. After so many failed attempts, many gave up, and a lot died out of drug complication.

The society always accuses high crime rate and various social vices emanating from slum and ghetto communities, but the question is whether these so-called ghetto youths enjoy doing crimes. Have they deliberately chosen this pattern of lives for themselves, or are they too lazy to work and make a better living? Were they too ambitious not to accept even a low-paid job or too arrogant not to engage in legal activities of life. Will they ever become productive if support and assistance are given to them? The fact is that our so-called street boys are not asking for much. All they were seeking for is a little to depend on in order to support life. The ghetto youths are not waste. There are so many brilliant and talented street boys. Most of them are crafty while many of them are talented artists. Talent is a blessing and a gift from God and does not depend on one's educational degree. Talent can be identified in the midst of intelligence.

Our street children are wise and calculative. They can do better if the government is willing to support them. They will become responsible for their own community development. The government must learn how to assemble the youths on the street, have a talk with them and identify their respective talents, and device a means to transform and build these talents for the development of the society. The unemployed youths on the street can actually work with their local government security service to ensure adequate community policing. The youths on the street who do not have any means of making a living could be locally employed to work with their community social welfare department to ensure proper environmental sanitation. Engaging the youths in petty jobs can equally help to set their mind off crime. This method is called 'working for the youths with the youths'.

Generally, there is an unemployment explosion in Africa. Despite the fact that about ten African countries account for the world's fastest growing economies, youth unemployment is increasing at an exponential rate. However, youth unemployment challenges in Africa are connected to youth population growth rate. There is an estimated 1.2 billion youths in the world between the ages of fifteen and twenty-four representing 17 per cent of the world's population. According to 2012 statistics, approximately 200 million people in Africa are between the ages of fifteen and twenty-four, while 40 per cent of the youths are globally unemployed.

There are numerous factors that contribute to the high rate of youth unemployment in Africa, such as inflexible labour market policy and regulation, insufficient establishment of manufacturing industries, and strategic employment pattern practised in many sectors. It is obvious to say that many African employers would rather employ a jobseeker with years of work experience, neglecting graduates with fresh skills and talents. This system is not helpful and does not support economic growth. Graduates must be given an opportunity to deploy the skills and knowledge they have acquired in school in the economic marketplace.

In Africa, the progress in the manufacturing sector is at a historical low. Overdependence on foreign goods is destroying the African economy. Africa must curtail excessive importation. If African government can plan, budget, and assemble the right materials and resources needed for production, within a decade, African youth with their potential can manufacture almost half of the goods being imported from Europe, Asia, and North America.

There is a need to undo the mentality that all foreign goods imported are standard and original made while goods produced in Africa are less superior. In order to meet up with the millennium development goals, African nations have to establish more manufacturing industries and strengthen the weakness in the existing ones so as to create jobs for the African youth. We must learn how to value and appreciate what we produce in our homes. This is one key strategy that China has used to boost their economy over the past ten years. It is said that one out of ten families in China engages in production, and this has helped to cut down the unemployment rate.

The consequences of youth unemployment are often linked to political unrest, delinquencies, and anti-social behaviour. There is poor economic growth due to productivity loss, lost income-tax revenues, and wasted capacities. Excluding young people from the labour market results in innovation declination. It means there is a lack of creativity and divergent thinking, which young people naturally possess. The African governments have to promote talents and invest in the future of the youths. Education is quite scarce among African youths. An estimated 133 million African youths are illiterate, and this figure makes up about 50 per cent of the total youth population. Vocational training is helping to bring young people back. Vocational education and training should be part of political programmes to combat youth unemployment. Creation of out-of-school youth development programmes is encouraged. It is necessary to prepare young people for an entrepreneurship culture, thereby empowering them to take their future into their hands. The government must help to modify the mindset of letting them realize their values. There is a huge benefit in cultivating entrepreneur mentality among young people. The youth could create enterprise as a means to find and create new jobs. It is noted that small and medium enterprises have created 33 per cent of the jobs over the last ten years and have helped to sustain the growth of the private sector.

There are other complex factors affecting different West African institutions. Some West African governments still practise the same old approach to management, which does not trigger development—the bondage of dependence and reliance on foreign aid. African nations have been enjoying independence for decades now, but most countries are still dependent on the former colonizers for assistance and decision-making. African leaders must deliberate the potential to transform the fortune present in the African continent. The leaders must focus their attention to create a welcoming environment that attracts investment. African nations are advised to adopt the African Union Commission agenda on sustainability, which include action plan for transformative Africa, peace and security action plan, integration, development and cooperation, shared values, and strengthening of institutions and capacities.

Before the recent Ebola outbreak, West African nations had a number of issues challenging the health sector. Also, leadership and management, incompetence monitoring, and assessment and policy implementation were poor. In addition to this troubling fact, there were ineffective policies and planning being carried out by the medical institution which resulted in poor quality care in the public sector.

A condition of dire poverty existed in the most Ebola-affected countries before the recent outbreak worsened the scenario. The infrastructural damage brought by fourteen years of brutal wars in Liberia has been the major cause of the country's brain drain. The war was responsible for the death of an estimated 270,000 people, and it forced millions to flee the country in search of refuge in the diaspora. The destruction of hydro-plants, hospitals, big investments, and private and commercial buildings by the rebels brought a share of extreme poverty and unemployment. The disaster also has a set of implications on the medical sector. Before the outbreak of the Liberian civil war, Liberia had an estimated 1,200 medical doctors but it was left with less than 100 medical doctors after the war. The economic consequence has seen Liberia GDP falling by over 90 per cent between 1987 and 1985.

However, it is important to draw a parallel between natural enrichment of African countries and the predicament befalling them at the same time. Africa is wealthy in oil, gas, iron, aluminium, and metals; African continent contains over one-third of the earth's cobalt. South Africa alone has 40 per cent of earth's gold supply, and Nigeria supplies about 50 per cent of US oil reserve. These are countries of fabulous wealth but whose people are living in grinding poverty. Liberia is rich in timber, rubber, and gold. Guinea is rich in aluminium ores and other minerals while Sierra Leone has plenty of diamonds, gold, cocoa beans, and titanium. These resources are developed by multinational corporations, extracted by means of low-paid local labourers, and exported to the enrichment of the corporation. It is obvious to say that the bilateral trades between these countries are not balanced. The outcome of such large business deal is expected to boost the economic growth of the poor West African nations. Western corporations were keen to build physical and human infrastructure, but little or no interest is shown to set up a manufacturing sector. The bloody civil war which hit Liberia and Sierra Leone in 1990 deteriorated their health and education system. Guinea had 1 physician per 10,000 people. Sierra Leone had less than one. This figure is very poor when compared to socialist Cuba with 59 doctors per 10,000 people. Liberia and Guinea have about 3 hospital beds per 10,000 people, while Cuba has about 49 hospital beds per 10,000 people. Africa's health institution must adopt new strategic direction that could introduce equitable and sustainable access to a properly functional health system. Sub-Saharan Africa will not be able to reduce poverty and hunger and improve child and maternal health care to meet the UN Millennium Development Goals set a decade ago by the United Nations unless African and Western leaders do much more.

Today, Ebola virus disease has struck our medical system. The whole world has joined hands together to fight the battle. When the American government deployed military troops to West Africa to fight the Ebola virus, the entire world realized that the situation has spread out of control. Many had lost their lives to the virus outbreak due to the nations' weakness. The African nations, including the global world, were not prepared for such unexpected tragedy. The Ebola cases in the United States and United Kingdom clearly show that no surface of the earth is safe. The journey has just begun. We have seen the level of the world's development as of twenty-first century. If all the world-leading scientists, physicians, and biologists, after decades of research, could not provide a solution to Ebola virus, it clearly shows human limitation at this stage of his life. The former generation knew that a tormenting season could hit the human race in his later life and thus had sent forth the same message to the later generation to better be aware and prepared. This is a preview of the future of humanity, one among many unknown natural disasters and pestilence that may war against humanity in the coming centuries.

The Ebola virus disease is here to disgrace us. It is high time we come together as one people and confront the challenges before us. It is our collective obligations to make our nation safe for us to dwell in. The world is at a crucial stage. Unexpected is happening. Our health is our wealth, our pride, and our future. We all need to admit the fact and face the reality. The nature of Ebola epidemics clearly shows that the race of mankind is subjected to a threat. Presently, the entire world is scared of Ebola mutating into an airborne disease (Ebola Reston) because that is the worst of it all. It kills at mass scale without recognizing personality or status. Although the possibility still remains very low, the world has to increase research and be prepared at all time. The African leaders should make health issues a priority and must create new programmes that will fast-track public health improvement.

A healthy nation is a wealthy nation.

5 Ebola Virus Disease: A Biowarfare Agent?

Introduction to Biowarfare

Biological warfare (BW), also known as germ warfare, is the use of biological toxins or infectious agents, such as bacteria, viruses, and fungi, with the intent to kill or incapacitate humans, animals, or plants as an act of war. Biological weapons (often termed *bio-weapons*, *biological threat agents*, or *bio-agents*) are organisms or replicating entities (viruses, which are not universally considered 'alive') that reproduce or replicate within their host victims. Entomological (insect) warfare is also considered a type of biological weapon. This type of warfare is distinct from nuclear warfare and chemical warfare. Together they make up nuclear, biological, and chemical warfare or weapons (NBC). All of these are considered *weapons of mass destruction* (WMDs). None of these fall under the term conventional weapons, which are primarily effective due to their destructive potential.

Biological weapons may be employed in various ways to gain a strategic or tactical advantage over the enemy, either by threats or by actual deployments. Like some of the chemical weapons, biological weapons may also be useful as area denial weapons. These agents may be lethal or non-lethal and may be targeted against a single individual, a group of people, or even an entire population. They may be developed, acquired, stockpiled, or deployed by nation states or by non-national groups. In the latter case or if a nation-state uses it clandestinely, it may also be considered bioterrorism. The advent of the germ theory and advances in bacteriology brought a new level of sophistication to the theoretical use of bio-agents in war. Biological sabotage in the form of anthrax and ganders was undertaken on behalf of the imperial German government during World War I (1914–1918) with indifferent results. The Geneva Protocol of 1925 prohibited the use of chemical weapons and biological weapons.

Bioterrorism

Bioterrorism is a criminal act against unsuspecting civilians using pathogenic biological agents, such as biological warfare agents. Bioterror and biological warfare agents are most often colourless, by and large odourless microorganisms (bacteria, viruses, fungi), or toxins (usually protein toxins) derived from microorganisms that can be spread in air as aerosols or in food or drink to infect as many people as possible. They are easily concealed and thus difficult to detect before the attack. In the aftermath of the events of September and October 2001, there was a heightened concern that the Ebola virus might be used as an agent of bioterrorism. Most people may argue that the deliberate release of Ebola virus is evidence of bioterrorism. The Centers for Disease Control and Prevention calls the Ebola virus a Category A agent. Category A agents are believed to present the greatest potential threat for harming public health and have high potential for large-scale dissemination. The public is generally more aware of Category A agents, and broad-based public health preparedness efforts are necessary. Other Category A agents include anthrax, plague, botulism, tularaemia, and smallpox.

Depolutation Agenda

The mythology surrounding the depopulation of the earth requires an attention. The misconception that the 'unworthy people' have to be eliminated in order to conserve energy and earth's resources for the members of the master race, who are qualified for existence, has heightened public concern. Before the recent Ebola outbreak in Africa, a lot of rumours were circulating about 90 per cent depopulation scheme plotted by world political leaders and global elites.

The outbreak of Ebola in the western region has given rise to such rumours and misconception over again. People were merging the outbreak with depopulation agenda. Some believed that this is one of the ways the world decision-makers intended to reduce the number of humans on earth. This implies that population reduction through biowarfare will achieve an immediate result on the Third World countries due to the weak medical system. Today, we face a global threat of malnutrition, overpopulation, lack of resources, pollution, a disturbed ecology, and nuclear weapon. The great experiment in consciousness of human evolution now stands on a precipice of its own making. The same consciousness which struggled for millions of years to ensure human survival is now on the verge of depleting its planet's resources, rendering its environment uninhabitable. At the present time, 15 million to 20 million people die each year of malnutrition and related causes; another 600 million are chronically hungry, and billions live in poverty without adequate shelter, education, or medical care.

The award-winning scientist Eric Pianca expressed his view on population reduction, saying:

> War and famine would not do. Instead, disease offered the most efficient and fastest way to kill the billions that must soon die if the population crisis is to be solved. AIDS is not an efficient killer because it is too slow. My favorite candidate for eliminating 90 per cent of the world's population is airborne Ebola (Ebola Reston), because it is both highly lethal and it kills in days, instead of years. We've got airborne diseases with 90 per cent mortality in humans. Think about that. You know, the bird flu's good, too. For everyone who survives, he will have to bury nine.

The depopulation agenda is being legitimized in print by various global *think tank* groups as a means to de-industrialize the planet in order to save it from the overuse of fossil fuels. Further, the depopulation agenda is being used as an excuse to protect the planet's inhabitants from a dwindling food source. The remaining question is, how far are the global elites willing to go to carry out their depopulation goals? According to Henry Kissinger, 'Depopulation should be the highest priority of foreign policy towards the third world'.

In 1939, T4 euthanasia programme was initiated in Nazi Germany during Adolf Hitler's rule. The general effort of T4 programme was to carefully eliminate the incurable sick, including physically and mentally disabled people. These people were considered useless eaters. They do not add value to the society and are causing shortage of the earth's resources. T4 programme intended to show pity to the helpless unfit by offering them death assistance. Though the programme was officially discontinued in 1941, the programme was already accounted for the death of estimated 85,000 sick people killed through starvation and lethal injection. T4 programme argues that the fund allocated for the care of criminals and insane people can best be used on the important development project.

The forced sterilization of Indian women in 1970 is one drastic method taken to cut down population growth in Asia. Bangladesh and Indonesia were also forced to have fewer children. This collective effort centred on childbirth regulation seeks to introduce a definite balance between population growth and limited resource supply. The theme of the United Nations First World Population Conference held in 1974 addressed overpopulation issues, to initiate a programme that outlines various population control measures, and to devise a quick means to tackle rapid population growth throughout. China is leading the step through their one-child policy.

In order to fulfil Margaret Sanger's desire on population reduction, which states that the most merciful thing that a large family does to one of its infant members is to kill it, in order to achieve this desire, a more radical method has to be involved. It is necessary to maintain human population rate in an average of 2.1 children per woman across the planet, but the question is often if the proposed standard could be basically maintained across all countries. In order to achieve the balance between population growth and consumption pattern, the government and the world decision-makers must match words with action. There is a need to implement strong and effective birth regulation policy. The role of Agenda 21 is to empower women to gain equal access to employment opportunities; this could reduce childbirth and reduce the birth rate.

The UN and the world leaders have given women more access to birth control, abortion, and frequent use of contraceptives to prevent pregnancy. The means proposed to combat population rise, such as several birth control measures, seems slow. For rapid change in population, the elites who desire quick result in population reduction may introduce more deadly options involving war and diseases. The centralized theme of depopulation project is to save the planet from collapse and man-made climate change, such as global warming. The elites believe that overpopulation and overuse of fossil fuel are causing the planet to run out of resources that sustain the ecosystem.

The rumour of depopulation by genocide has attracted suspicion and accusations by local populations in Liberia and Sierra Leone, the epicentre of Ebola outbreak in West Africa. A lot of angry protesters were laying accusation that the bio-weapon lab in Kenema, Sierra Leone, is spreading Ebola virus and the global elites continue spending billions of dollars in funding bio-weapon laboratories. The sudden death of Glenn Thomas, a consultant to the World Health Organization in Geneva, an expert in Ebola and AIDS virus who was flying aboard the Malaysia Airline Boeing 777 in July 2014, has also generated much controversy supporting their claim.

Glenn Thomas was one of the spokesmen for the World Health Organization and participated in a series of investigations into testing operations with the Ebola virus in the laboratory of biological weapons in Kenema Hospital in Sierra Leone. The rumor claimed that Thomas had refused to participate in the cover-up of a revealing evidence showing that the diagnostic lab had manipulated to give positive diagnosis for Ebola, and this could be the reason Glenn Thomas was murdered.

New Israeli Virus Bio-Weapon Targets Arabs Only

There is a development of bio-weapons designed to kill only designated races and ethnic groups, such as racial bomb. It was reported in the *London Sunday Times* in 1997 that Israel was working on a biological weapon which is genetically targeted against Arabs. At the same time, the Israeli scientists used South African genetic warfare research in an attempt to develop an *ethnic bullet*.

Israeli scientists at the super-secret Nes Ziona biowarfare laboratory near Tel Aviv have engineered deadly microorganisms that only attack DNA within the cells of victims with distinctive Arab genes. Nes Ziona produces a wide range of chemical and biological weapons that is reportedly larger than all Arab and Iranian biowarfare laboratories combined. The Israeli research mirrors biological studies conducted by South African scientists during the apartheid era and disclosed in testimony before the Truth and Reconciliation Commission. Daan Goosen, head of a South African chemical and biological warfare facility, said that his team was ordered in the 1980s to develop a *pigmentation weapon* to target only black people. The British Medical Association has become so concerned about the lethal potential of genetically based biological weapons and, as such, has opened an investigation.

Allegations of Weaponized Virus

During the same time frame, but buried behind the scenes, HIV and Ebola appeared in the same region of Africa for the first time and at the same time. HIV swept across much of Africa, decimating a large swath of the population. Some African communities had as many as 90 per cent of the adults die from the disease in some villages and towns. This accusation always refers to the adoption of UN Agenda 21 population reduction policies being put in place and the signing of an executive order by the America government in order to exercise power to begin rounding up American citizens' respiratory system against their will. This is something that is not clear and has attracted public concern to the possibility of such accusation. However, looking at a significant number of depopulation scheme put in place, there are still more question than answers relating to depopulation by genocide and Ebola outbreak. There is a myth that Ebola will hit the American border through the unprotected southern border. The prime suspects are an untold number of West Africans, estimated at 100,000 in Central America, streaming into the country as drug couriers. These immigrants are suspected to have come from the Ebola-affected regions in the West Africa.

Overpopulation Is a Myth

The anticipation that the depopulation of the earth will save the planet from a sudden collapse is seen as a mythology by large members of the public. Many argue that industrialization, increase in production, and employment opportunities are the only means to adjust birth rate and slow down population growth throughout the world.

Presently, the birth rate declines dramatically in Italy and the United States. The birth rate is 1.4 in Italy and 1.8 in the United States. These figures show evidence of a highly industrialized country. In order to achieve balance between the ecosystem and the inhabitants, population growth has to be contained through a well-planned policy.

The global government should reconduct a research on climate change to actually find out if overpopulation is the root cause of global warming and to observe if the planet is really running out of fossil fuel, bringing about ecological damage.

6 ZMapp: Reaction from the West

ZMapp is an experimental biopharmaceutical drug comprising three humanized monoclonal antibodies under development as a treatment for Ebola virus disease. The drug was first tested in humans during the 2014 West African Ebola virus outbreak. The ZMapp drug is being developed by Mapp Biopharmaceutical Inc. It is a result of the collaboration between Mapp Biopharmaceutical (San Diego), LeafBio (the commercial arm of Mapp Biopharmaceutical), Defyrus Inc. (Toronto), the US government, and the Public Health Agency of Canada. The antibody work came out of research projects funded by the US Army more than a decade ago and years of funding by the Public Health Agency of Canada. ZMapp is composed of three humanized monoclonal antibodies (mAbs) that combine the best components of MB-003 (Mapp) and ZMAb (Defyrus/PHAC), each of which were combinations of mAbs. Two of the mAbs in ZMapp were taken from ZMAb and one of them came from MB-003.

In 2014, Samaritan's Purse worked with the FDA and Mapp Biopharmaceutical to make the drug available for two of its health workers that were infected by Ebola during their work in Liberia under the expanded access programme. At the time, there were only a few doses of ZMapp in existence. According to the Samaritan's Purse, Kent Brantly received the first dose of ZMapp nine days after falling ill. Brantly received a blood transfusion from a fourteen-year-old boy who survived an Ebola virus infection before being treated with the ZMapp serum. Nancy Writebol, working alongside Brantly, was also treated with Zmapp. The condition of both health workers improved, especially in Brantly's case, before being transported back to the United

States. Emory University Hospital specialized in Ebola treatment. Writable and Brantly were released from the hospital on 21 August 2014.

The West African nation of Liberia, which was affected by the 2014 outbreak, had secured enough ZMapp to treat three Liberians with the Ebola virus. One of the three to receive the drug, Dr Abraham Borbor, a Liberian doctor and deputy chief physician at Liberia's largest hospital, also died in 25 August 2014. William Pooley, a British male nurse who contracted Ebola while working in Sierra Leone, was also treated with ZMapp in August 2014. Mapp announced on 11 August 2014 that its supplies of the drug had been exhausted. Nigerian authorities had requested the experimental ZMapp drug from the US Centers for Disease Control and Prevention to combat the Ebola virus, which was fast claiming a growing number of lives across the West African nations, but the US government cited a shortage of drugs. The lack of drugs and unavailability of experimental treatment in the most affected regions have spurred some controversy.

On 6 August 2014, Peter Piot, who co-discovered the Ebola virus, and other scientists, including the director of the Wellcome Trust, called for the release of ZMapp for affected African nations. The fact that the drug has been given to Americans and European but not sufficient to serve Africans has provoked outrage, feeding into African perceptions of Western insensitivity and arrogance with a deep sense of mistrust and betrayal still lingering over the exploitation and abuses of the colonial era.

However, on the response to this outbreak, numerous organizations and countries have rendered an immense support and contributions to fight this virus disease.

Response by Organisations and Foundations

World Health Organisation

The office of the World Health Organization is leading the fight against Ebola virus. WHO declared the outbreak an International Public Health Emergency on 8 August 2014 and has delivered effective support to contain the outbreak.

On 25 August, WHO announced that it had sent protective equipment to medical staff in the Democratic Republic of the Congo.

On 28 August, WHO announced that it is seeking 490 million dollars to fund the fight against the outbreak.

United State Centers for Disease Control and Prevention (CDC)

At the same time, the CDC was working together with WHO, Médecins Sans Frontières (Doctors without Borders), and many other institutions and non-government organization to combat the outbreak. By 26 August, the CDC had issued a Level 3 travel warning for Sierra Leone, Liberia, and Guinea, and a Level 2 travel warning for Nigeria. The purpose of issuing this warning is to ensure active precaution that will prevent imported cases.

World Bank Group

As of April 2015, the World Bank Group has mobilized finance at the tune of 1.62 billion US dollars to help Ebola response on the hardest-hit countries.

African Development Bank

The financial support from the African Development Bank reaches 220 million US dollars.

African Union

The African Union launched an urgent initiative to recruit more health workers from among its members following the complaint received by the World Health Organization. By the end of August 2014, WHO reported that too many losses of health workers had made it difficult for them to provide sufficient foreign medical personnel.

European Union

The European Commission showed their sympathy towards this virulent outbreak and pledged their support; in an effort to combat Ebola virus, the European Union spent a total of 1.3 billion euros.

Economic Community of West Africa States (ECOWAS)

By the end of March 2014, the Economic Community of West Africa States donated 250,000 US dollars to fight the Ebola virus outbreak during the forty-fourth summit of head of states and African government. Furthermore, ECOWAS Commission and African Development Bank had signed Grant Protocol Agreement worth 3 million US dollars for the coordination of the Ebola crisis response project.

United Nations Children's Emergency Fund (UNICEF)

UNICEF established 200-million-US-dollar programmes as part of their Ebola response aid.

Médecins Sans Frontières

The humanitarian aid organization also known as Doctors without Borders has been in the frontline of Ebola outbreak emergency response. MSF had set up multiple health centres and provided health equipment to three most affected countries and at the same time deployed about 676 health personnel to care for the sick people.

International Federation of Red Cross and Red Cross Crescent Societies

The International Federation of Red Cross and Red Cross Crescent Societies had budgeted more than 100 million Swiss francs to fight the epidemic, also built treatment unit in Kenema, Sierra Leone, the epicentre of the outbreak.

Innovative Medicines Initiative

The innovative medicines initiative launched a total of eight budgets to the amount of 215 million euros in January 2015 to aid vaccine development for Ebola treatment.

Samaritan's Purse

The Christian charity showed a committed effort in response to the outbreak and also worked with other non-government group to provide direct medical care in different locations in Liberia.

Wellcome Trust

On 23 August, Wellcome Trust pledged support of 3.2 million pounds to speed up Ebola vaccine trials.

Global Alliance for Vaccine and Immunization

GAVI, the Global Alliance for the Vaccine and Immunization, had established a special vaccine task force for new vaccine development at the cost of approximately 300 million US dollars.

World Food Programme (WFP)

The World Food Programme organized a programme plan that mobilized food aid for remote areas of the affected regions.

Food and Agriculture Organization

The United Nations' Food and Agriculture Organization launched a 30-million-US-dollar campaign programme to ensure food and nutrition security.

International Charter on Space and Major Disaster

The International Charter on Space and Major Disaster carried out its first epidemiological role in 9 October 2014 to monitor an outbreak in Sierra Leone.

United States Agency for International Development (USAID)

The United States Agency for International Development deployed more health workers in West Africa to help run the Ebola treatment centres.

International Medical Corps

The International Medical Corps is working in Liberia and Sierra Leone to conduct safe burial practices.

Direct Relief

The Direct Relief organization had deployed 100 tons of medical supply valued at 6 million US dollars to the Ebola hit region.

Oxfam

The charity organization Oxfam is helping to provide hygiene and sanitation equipment to Ebola treatment centres and boosting mass publication about the disease. Oxfam also announced that it is seeking to raise funds of at least 25 million pounds to prevent 3.2 million people at risk of catching the virus.

Goal

The charity organization is delivering community sensitization and information in Sierra Leone.

Bill and Melinda Gates Foundation

The Gates Foundation donated 50 million US dollars to the UN and 2 million dollars to the CDC to counter the outbreak.

Paul G. Allen Family Foundation

Paul G. Allen Family Foundation donated 2.8 million US dollars to the Red Cross in August 2014 and also pledged 10 million US dollars to the United States Centers for Disease Control and Prevention.

Dangote Foundation

Dangote Foundation pledged the sum of 3 million US dollars to support Ebola response and had already donated almost 1 million US dollars to national Ebola fight in Nigeria.

Mark Zuckerberg and Family

Facebook founder and CEO, Mark Zuckerberg, and his wife, Dr Priscilla Chan, made a grant of 25 million US dollars through United States Centers for Disease Prevention and Control. The grant will be used to fund Ebola fight in Sierra Leone, Liberia, and Guinea.

Response by Countries

Australia
Australian government pledged to donate 1 million US dollars to the World Health Organization to help fight the Ebola outbreak.

Morocco
By April 2014, Morocco has increased medical surveillance at Casablanca Airport, a regional hub for flights moving to and from Africa regions.

Canada
As of August 2014, Canadian government had donated resources worth 5,195,000 US dollars to both humanitarian and public health interventions to support Ebola response action. The resources include doses of untested Ebola virus vaccine donated to the World Health Organization.

Nigeria
Nigerian government donated 500,000 US dollars to support Liberia battles outbreak and also sent teams of volunteer medical workers. At the same time, the president of the Federal Republic of Nigeria, Goodluck Jonathan, also made a donation to Guinea, Sierra Leone, the West African Health Organization (WHAO), and the ECOWAS Pool Fund against Ebola, totalling 3.5 million US dollars.

Japan
As of August 2014, the government of Japan had donated over 2 million dollars to WHO, UNICEF, and the Red Cross Societies to help contain the outbreak.

Togo

Togo had set up more than 13,000 active volunteers in cooperation with the Togo Red Cross Society for the preparation of an unexpected outbreak in Togo.

Brazil

Following the request for international cooperation made by the World Health Organization, the health ministry of Brazil donated 1.2 tons of supplies of antibiotics, anti-inflammatories, gloves, and masks.

South Africa

South African government in cooperation with the country's leading companies and donors had pledged services, goods, and cash valued at 12 million rands to support Ebola-hit countries. Also, the South African immigration authorities had increased surveillance and screening of all travellers returning from Guinea, Liberia, and Sierra Leone.

Cuba

Following the extraordinary Ebola summit held in Havana on 20 October 2014, the government of Cuba announced that it would send more than three hundred medical workers to Ebola-stricken countries, adding to the 165 workers that had already been sent to Sierra Leone. The Ebola outbreak response support from Cuba motivates other international communities to step up their commitment towards containing the outbreak.

United States of America

United States is leading into Ebola response funding with the commitment of over 300 million US dollars, sending troops to West Africa and setting up multiple health centres across the Ebola-hit countries.

Russia
Russia pledged a support of 19 million US dollars to support research and humanitarian aid project.

Netherlands
The Dutch government pledged over 38-million-euro support to help fight the Ebola epidemic in West Africa and deployed naval ships carrying medical supplies to West Africa.

United Kingdom
The British government had unveiled 201.25-million-US-dollar action plan (equivalent to 125 million British pounds) to aid Ebola emergency response.

China
The Chinese government pledged an estimated 34-million-US-dollar aid to West African countries and international organizations fighting the outbreak. Chinese scientists continued Ebola virus experimental drug trials and also sent supplies of medical protectives, thermal detectors, and disinfectants to Sierra Leone and Guinea.

New Zealand
New Zealand pledged about 397,000 US dollars to the World Health Organization.

Germany
Germany gave 13.37 million US dollars to the World Health Organization.

Ghana
Ghana hosts the UN Mission for Ebola Emergency Response. The Ghanaian government offered Accra as a support base to help fight Ebola in the neighbouring countries.

Timor-Leste
Timor-Leste had pledged 1 million US dollars to West Africa's regional response unit.

Philippines
The Philippine government withdrew its 115 UN peacekeepers working in Guinea to minimize the risk posed by larger outbreak.

Saudi Arabia
On 1 April 2014, Saudi Arabia imposed travel ban on Muslims travelling from Liberia, Sierra Leone, and Guinea. The Arab government had stop issuing visa to those going to Mecca from Ebola-affected countries.

Ivory Coast
Ivory Coast closed its borders to the neighbouring countries.

Equatorial Guinea
Equatorial Guinea had cancelled all regional flights and stopped issuing visas to the affected countries till further notice.

Kenya
The government of Kenya had banned people travelling from Liberia, Sierra Leone, and Guinea from entering all ports. Kenya also pledged 1 million US dollars to support Ebola regional response.

Egypt
Egypt had delivered over 3,000 tons of medical supplies to be distributed to the affected countries.

Qatar

Qatar had placed bans on food and animal importation from Liberia, Sierra Leone, Guinea, and Nigeria.

Malaysia

Malaysia planed to send tons of medical supplies to the affected region.

Israel

The Israeli government had sent six cargos containing medical supplies and had contributed about 8.75 million US dollars for Ebola emergency response.

France

France, in cooperation with the French Red Cross Society, had pledged up to 89 million US dollars, including a plan to set up an Ebola treatment centre in Guinea.

Norway

Norway made a pledge of 23 million US dollars to the World Health Organization and different non-government organizations to help battle Ebola outbreak.

Ethiopia

In October 2014, Ethiopia donated 500,000 US dollars to the Ebola-affected countries.

India

India donated 10 million US dollars to UN Mission for Ebola Emergency Response (UNMEER).

Reactions from Airlines

28 July 2014
Arik Air suspended flights into Liberia and Sierra Leone to prevent Ebola virus outbreak in Nigeria.

11 August 2014
Ghana banned flights from Liberia, Nigeria, Sierra Leone, and Guinea.

11 August 2014
Ivory Coast imposed a ban on flights to and from Sierra Leone, Liberia, and Guinea.

14 August 2014
Korean Air had announced to suspend flights to and from Kenya.

27 August 2014
British Airways suspended flights to or from Sierra Leone and Liberia till 2015.

7 The Fear and Stigma of Ebola Virus

The breaking of news of the 2014 Ebola virus outbreak in West Africa and its rapid circulation from one region to another, affecting multiple people at a time, hit the global world with an immense surprise and had left a lot of people in fear and panic, considering the high mortality rate of the illness and consequent outbreak since 1976, when Ebola virus was first discovered. This poses a huge threat to global health, but there is a need to approach this in a mature and responsible way without sentiment. Human discrimination and avoidance of person-to-person interaction made it difficult to fight the outbreak. The reaction from international communities' closing airlines and placing a travel ban on Ebola-affected countries is quite unfriendly; more so, the idea of some African countries with no Ebola cases closing their borders against Ebola victim countries is highly unethical.

Although avoiding direct contact with people carrying the Ebola virus is one of the key measures used to reduce the spread of the disease, this also has negative effect as people who suffer from other severe illnesses like malaria are sometimes admitted into isolation as precaution. But in most cases, even when they passed their incubation period and got discharged, the community still believes they were actually being treated for Ebola and could still be contagious. Due to the fear of being marginalized or isolated, a lot of people chose to conceal their illness.

The public panic and social unrest have widely affected international business appointments and social interactions. Some foreign countries indicated their selfishness in protecting their own citizens by declaring off-travel chances to all affected regions in an attempt to prevent imported outbreak.

International business projects and contracts undergoing execution before the Ebola virus outbreak have been suspended due to travel ban and airline closure. This has widely affected the forecast of economic growth on a very slow lane.

Ebola stigmatization is on the rise. The victims are isolated, and their latest contact is traced and quarantined. Ebola virus reshapes one's mindset towards other people; it threatens the peace and unity which exist among people. It introduces a new form of unintended hatred that is practised without a choice. Since Ebola can be transmitted through blood or bodily fluid of an infected person, health personnel and medical troops totally banned anyone from coming close to an Ebola patient. Loved ones die without saying farewell to their beloved. Business functions and growth are very slow at the time of the outbreak. The whole world is suffering from the economic downturn, but the current outbreak of Ebola virus disease makes it worst. Countries have channelled the energies which are needed to combat economic crisis towards fighting the spread of Ebola virus disease.

What about the medical department? Health workers resign from their duties due to the fear of contracting the Ebola virus. Some hospitals refuse to admit sick patients that are brought at emergency without undergoing a primary test to examine the nature of sickness due to fear of Ebola virus. I was called that a friend slumped and was rushed to the nearest clinic only to discover that the hospital management refused to admit him without conducting an initial diagnosis. They were referred to the general hospital simply because they suspected Ebola case, but before they could get to the general hospital, the sick young man gave up the ghost as they had to battle excessive traffic on the highway. The fear of Ebola virus has taken away the life of the helpless young man. The autopsy showed that the person died out of stress and blood shortage.

The fear of Ebola virus disease is causing hardship and is reducing the standard of living of many people. There is ongoing mass starvation due to disruptions in food trade and marketing in the three West African countries most affected by Ebola. This has made food increasingly expensive and hard to come by. Labour shortages are putting the upcoming harvest season at serious risk. In Guinea, Liberia, and Sierra Leone, quarantine zones and restrictions on people's movement have negatively curtailed the movement and marketing of food. This led to panic buying, food shortages, and significant food price hikes on some commodities.

Especially in urban centres, butchers are bitterly complaining that the fear of an Ebola virus outbreak has put them off business as there is little or no demand for meat at the time of this uncontrollable outbreak as unconfirmed rumours are circulating that bush animals are the primary reservoir of Ebola virus. Irrespective the global effort in combating the outbreak, it seems the progress is slow. This has become the people's most pressing concern, and many are asking if the world is losing the battle in containing the outbreak. The major purpose is to curb fear and stigma by helping people to avoid panicking. That is why it is important to create a communication network by providing life-saving information to communities so they better will understand the disease and know how to protect themselves.

Survivors of Ebola also suffer from stigma. Even after they have fully recovered and have been discharged, the community still reject them, believing they are still harmful. They do not want them in the market, in their house, or places of worship. Families who were affected must get proper treatment, but after they have recovered and are declared free of the virus, they still need community's support to return to normal life. This is one of the messages that the Red Cross volunteers are giving to the communities.

The facts and fictions associated with an Ebola outbreak make people unsettled across Africa. Prominent people fled to foreign countries with their families on the Ebola virus prevention trip. This literally means that if everyone ultimately secures a way to escape from West Africa due to the fear of Ebola virus, 'we shall come back in later years to see the nation dominated by unseen vampires'.

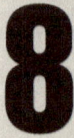

8 Graph of Ebola Virus Facts and Fictions and Infection Timeline (1976–2014)

The latest outbreak in humans represents not just the most recent but also the most deadly among several incidents dating back to 1976.

Initial Ebola Outbreak in Central Africa (1976)
The hemorrhagic fever from the Ebola virus first occurred in two simultaneous outbreaks in Zaire (now called the Democratic Republic of the Congo, or DRC) and Sudan. In Yambuku, Zaire, it killed 280 people. The disease was first thought to be a Marburg virus, but it was identified later that year as a different but related disease. It is named after the Ebola River, which is near the outbreak site.

Initial Outbreak in Sudan (1976)
The outbreak in Nzara, Sudan, killed 151 people and infected 284.

Researcher Accidentally Contaminated Self (1976)
A researcher accidentally sticks himself with a contaminated needle containing the Sudanese version of the virus. He survives and the disease does not spread.

Second Sudanese Outbreak (1979)
A second outbreak in Nzara at the same site as the 1976 outbreak killed twenty-two of the thirty-four infected people.

Gabon Outbreak in Mining Camp (1994)

Ebola exploded in a gold mining camp and killed thirty-one people. Officials thought the culprit was yellow fever but later identified it as Ebola.

Major Outbreak Hit Hospitals in Zaire (1995)

A large outbreak in Zaire spread through hospitals, killing 250 of 315 infected.

Tainted Chimpanzee Infected Thirty-Seven in Gabon (1996)

Nineteen people become sick after butchering an infected chimpanzee. The disease spread to family members, inflecting a total of thirty-seven people and killing twenty-one.

NIH Tested Vaccine (2000–2001)

A team of NIH scientists developed a vaccine tested on monkeys. It protected the primates from deadly doses of the virus.

Outbreak Claimed Ninety-Six in Gabon and the Republic of the Congo (October 2000–March 2002)

An outbreak crossed the border between Gabon and the Republic of the Congo. A total of 96 people died out of the 122 people infected.

Republic of the Congo Hit Once Again (December 2002–April 2003)

Another outbreak occurred, killing 128 people of the more than 143 infected.

Ebola Misdiagnosed as Measles in Sudan (2004)

A small outbreak infected seventeen people and killed seven in Yambio county, now part of South Sudan. Many of these cases were previously misdiagnosed as measles.

The Graph of Ebola Virus: Facts and Fictions

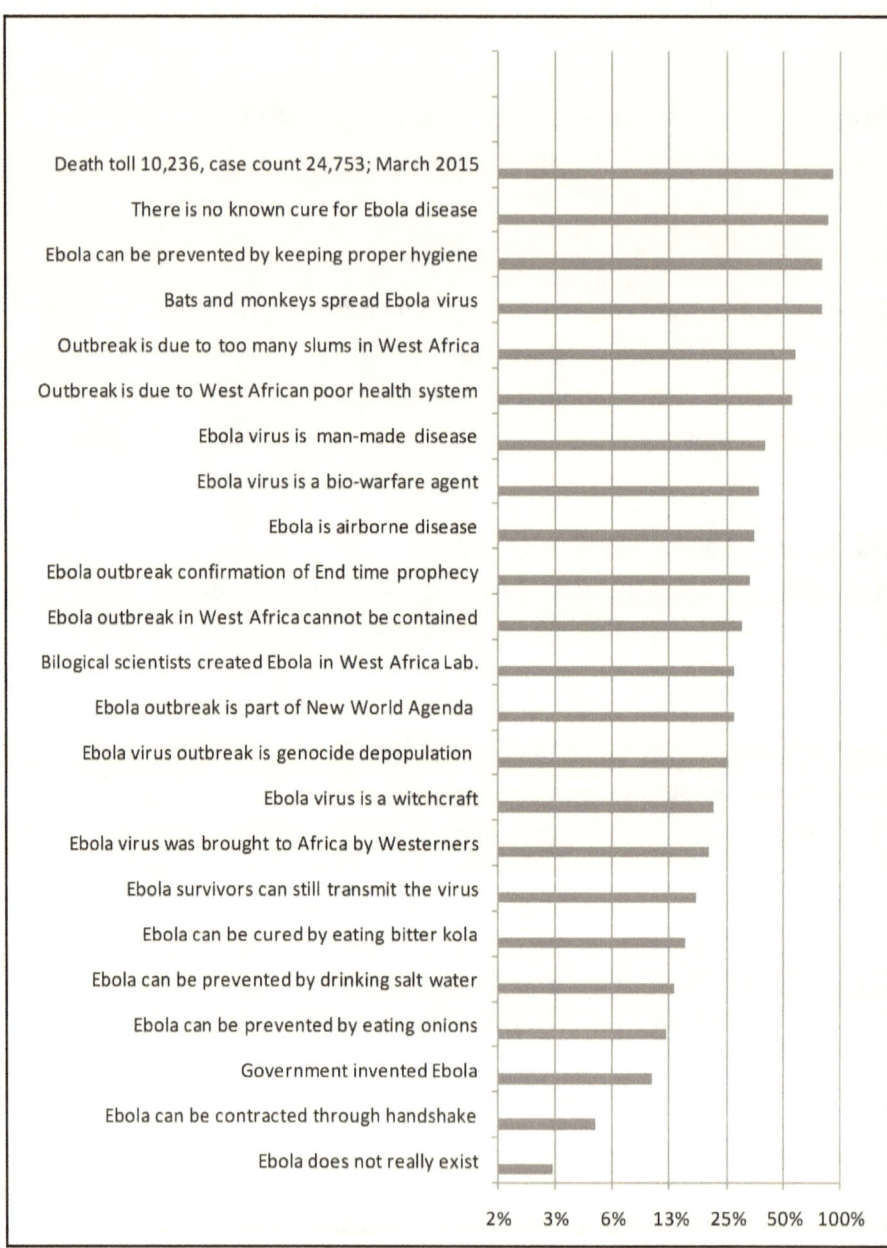

Number of people that believe.

Accidental Contamination in Russia (2004)
One person died after a laboratory contamination incident.

Outbreak in the Congo (2007)
A large outbreak occurred in Kasai-Occidental province, killing 187 of 264 infected.

New Ebola Strain Identified in Uganda (December 2007–January 2008)
The first outbreak of the new Ebola Bundibugyo strain was reported, infecting 149 and killing 37.

Key Protein Found to Help Combat Virus (July 2008)
Researchers identified a protein in the Ebola virus that could serve as a location for targeted treatment.

Congo Struck Once Again (December 2008–8 November 2009)
An outbreak killed fifteen of thirty-two people in Kasai-Occidental.

Virologist Contaminated (March 2009)
A German virologist accidentally pricked herself with a needle contaminated with Ebola but recovered.

Small Outbreak in Uganda (June 2012–October 2012)
The outbreak infected eleven people and killed four.

Bundibugyo Strain Infected Thirty-Six (June 2012–November 2012)

An outbreak of the Bundibugyo strain killed thirteen people and infected thirty-six. This outbreak has no relation to the contemporaneous event in Uganda.

Small Outbreak Killed Three More (November 2012–15 January 2013)

A small outbreak in Uganda infected six and killed three.

Cross-Border Ebola Outbreak Ebola Virus Hit West Africa (28 December 2013)

West Africa's first Ebola victim, a young Guinean boy, died.

Ebola Rapidly Evolving in Guinea (March 2014)

Guinea's Ministry of Health notified the World Health Organization of a 'rapidly evolving' Ebola outbreak. By that date, forty-nine cases were reported with twenty-nine deaths.

First Ebola Cases Reported in Liberia (30 March 2014)

Liberia reported its first two confirmed cases of Ebola from patients who had travelled to Guinea—one of whom, a thirty-five-year-old woman, died on 21 March.

Mali Suspected First Ebola Cases (7 April 2014)

Mali reported four suspected cases of Ebola virus, two of which had travelled from Guinea.

WHO Reported More Dead (10 April 2014)

WHO reported 101 deaths from the still-emerging outbreak in West Africa.

Bodies of Deceased Patients Spread Ebola to Family (25 May 2014)

Two Sierra Leone citizens died of Ebola in Guinea. Their bodies were repatriated to their country, where many family members then contracted the virus at their funerals.

WHO Reported Increasing Death Tolls (17 June 2014)

WHO reported 528 Ebola cases in West Africa, resulting in 337 deaths.

The Caseload Continues to Grow (7 July 2014)

WHO reported 844 sick and 518 deaths globally.

First Case Reported in Nigeria (25 July 2014)

Nigeria reported its first Ebola case carried in by a forty-year-old Liberian man. More cases appeared in Nigeria following the man's death from the disease, but the outbreak was ultimately contained.

Leader in Ebola Fight Died of Infection (29 July 2014)

Sierra Leone's Sheik Humarr Khan, a leader in the country's fight against the epidemic, succumbed to the disease.

US Aid Worker Contracted Ebola (2 August 2014)

US aid worker Kent Brantly tested positive for Ebola and was flown from West Africa to Emory University Hospital in Atlanta. He received treatment with the experimental drug ZMapp.

Second US Aid Worked Contracted Disease (5 August 2014)

A second American aid worker Nancy Writebol tested positive for Ebola and was evacuated for treatment at Emory.

Experimental Treatment Successful in US Aid Workers (21 August 2004)

Both Brantly and Writebol recovered and were released from Emory after being administered the drug ZMapp, which contains three different antibodies that derail replicating Ebola proteins. It remains unclear if the drug affected their recovery.

Patient Zero Believed to be Sole Source of Ebola Outbreak (29 August 2014)

Patient zero for the disease outbreak in Sierra Leone was identified in a paper published in science.

Blood Transfusions from Survivors Is the Best Way to Fight Ebola (5 September 2014)

WHO recommended using blood transfusions from patients who recovered from Ebola as best way to fight the disease.

WHO Projected Bleak Future (23 September 2014)

The World Health Organization released bleak projections for how bad the outbreak could get, potentially infecting 20,000 cases by November.

First Ebola Case in the United States (30 September 2014)

Texas Health Presbyterian Hospital in Dallas (THPH) announced it had in isolation the first case of Ebola in the US. The patient, Thomas Duncan, was a Liberian who flew to Texas.

Death Toll over 3,000 (30 September 2014)

WHO announced 6,574 cases globally, with 3,091 deaths.

NBC Cameraman Contracted the Disease (2 October 2014)

An NBC freelance cameraman Ashoka Mukpo contracted the virus in Liberia and was evacuated to the US for treatment.

First US Patient Died (8 October 2014)

Thomas Duncan died of Ebola at THPH after receiving brincidofovir, an antiviral drug.

American Nurse Contracted Virus (10 October 2014)

Nina Pham, a nurse who treated Thomas Duncan, contracted Ebola virus. She went into isolation at Texas Health Presbyterian Hospital in Dallas and then was transferred to Bethesda for treatment at an NIH facility.

A Second Nurse Contracted Virus (14 October 2014)

A second nurse who cared for Duncan, Amber Vinson, also contracted the virus. She entered THPH for treatment and was then transferred to Emory University Hospital in Atlanta.

WHO Declared Senegal Free from Ebola (17 October 2014)

The country only had one case, imported from Guinea.

Ebola Czar Appointed in US (17 October 2014)

President Obama appointed Ron Klain as Ebola czar.

Ebola Stopped in Nigeria (20 October 2014)

WHO declared Nigeria free from Ebola.

First Case Reported in NYC (23 October 2014)

New York City reported its first Ebola case—Craig Allen Spencer, a doctor who treated patients in Guinea. Spencer was rushed to Bellevue Hospital for diagnosis and treatment.

First Case Reported in Mali (23 October 2014)

Mali confirmed its first case of Ebola. The two-year-old girl was the only case in Mali but died the following day.

Nina Pham Released from Isolation (24 October 2014)

The NIH declared Nina Pham Ebola free and released her from isolation.

Over 10,000 Cases Reported (24 October 2014)

WHO reported 10,141 Ebola cases, of which 4,922 people had died.

US Aid Worker Detained in Newark, New Jersey (24 October 2014)

Nurse Kaci Hickox returned to the US from Sierra Leone, where she had been working as part of Doctors without Borders. After landing at Newark Liberty International Airport, she was questioned for six hours and forced to stay in an isolation tent at a nearby hospital for three days even though she has no symptoms of Ebola.

US Aid Worker Released to Maine (27 October 2014)

Hickox was allowed to drive home to Fort Kent, Maine. But there, officials tried to legally force her into mandatory quarantine.

Louisiana Pushed for Quarantine (27 October 2014)

Louisiana government officials stepped in to request that anyone who had been to Liberia, Sierra Leone, or Guinea in the past twenty-one days shall not attend the American Society of Tropical Medicine and Hygiene annual meeting being held in New Orleans starting on 2 November.

Liberia Caseload Dropping (29 October 2014)
WHO reported that Liberia appeared to be beating back Ebola. Its caseload, the organization said, may be dropping by as much as 25 per cent a week.

Kaci Hickox Defied Quarantine Order (30 October 2014)
In an act of defiance, Hickox went on an hour-long bike ride with her partner in her hometown.

Maine Judge Lifted Hickox Quarantine (31 October 2014)
A Maine judge ruled that Hickox could leave her home, but she would need to continue monitoring for a fever and alert officials about her travel plans.

FDA Unveiled Plans for Ebola Drugs (5 November 2014)
At the American Society of Tropical Medicine and Hygiene conference in Louisiana, federal officials from the US Food and Drug Administration unveiled plans to test multiple Ebola drugs simultaneously in a study that will involve a single comparison group. The approach, they say, will allow them to get faster answers about what drugs work against Ebola.

Monitoring Period for Dallas Staff Ended (7 November 2014)
The twenty-one-day monitoring period for those who were potentially exposed to Ebola patient Duncan ended without further cases developing. In total, 177 people, including health-care workers, household contacts and community members were monitored because of their potential exposure.

First US Treatment Unit Opened (10 November 2014)
The first Ebola treatment unit built and staffed with US government funding opened to receive its first patients on that week. More than 2,100 US civilian

and military personnel work in West Africa on the Ebola response, making it the largest-ever US response to a global health crisis.

New York Patient Released from Hospital (11 November 2014)

The first Ebola patient in New York City, Doctor Craig Allen Spencer, was released from the hospital after surviving the virus. He had spent nineteen days in the hospital after being diagnosed with the virus. At the hospital, he received a blood plasma transfusion from Ebola survivor Nancy Writebol. New York health officials monitored 357 people for potential exposure to Spencer, but the monitoring period for that ended Thursday, 1 November 2014.

Second Fatal Case in Mali (12 November 2014)

Government officials confirmed the country's second fatal case of Ebola virus disease, a nurse that cared for an Ebola patient at a private hospital in the capital Bamako. The case appeared to be linked to an imam from Guinea who died at the clinic in late October from kidney failure and was not tested for Ebola. Public health workers investigated other probable cases and tried to locate many mourners who attended the imam's funeral rites and ritual washing. Two additional cases were reported on 25 November.

9 Population Control Measures

The power of population is so superior to the power of the earth to produce subsistence for man. Premature death must in some shape or the other visit the human race; the vices of mankind are active and able ministers of depopulation. Thomas Robert Malthus expressed his concern about the rapid expansion of humanity.

Today, the world is challenged with a severe threat of global warming. The consequent rise in population over the past two decades has been accused to be the major cause of climate change. Famine and pollution are caused by human intervention, and only a change in human attitude can bring ultimate solution to these predicaments. In order to save the planet from an untimely collapse, the world's population control advocates are calling for population reduction and possible control.

The ambition to bring balance between the number of people present on earth and the available resources that sustain the ecosystem is as old as the earth itself. The world is already faced with economic decline and disturbed ecology. Futurists speculate that population explosion could add more damage, causing the planet to run out of fossil fuel.

Over the years, countless of population control programmes have been initiated, and human depopulation agenda has grown stronger even in more recent times. The general theme of these programmes and efforts is to maintain the human population at a reasonable figure. Certain measures set out to pursue this objective might be in some ways disastrous. The theory of depopulation by genocide has, however, become an acceptable platform to some ruling elites who desire quick change in human population.

It is to eliminate a large number of people through an act of war, abortion, forced sterilization, and control of the reproductive organs. The assumption that the inferior races produce disastrous breed and could not be allowed to reproduce has led to the initiation of more population control programmes centred on the elimination of the unfit, the disabled, mentally and physically challenged people and not limited to the elderly people. As for the populists, these people are seen as burdensome lives and deserve to die.

These objectives involve the segregation of the morons and the genetic sterilization of the inferior races, and to murder the handicapped through starvation and lethal injection. In addition to their effort, killer physicians might be instructed to withhold food and medical assistance to the sick victims. More so, withdrawal of charity is part of the strategy in order not to extend the lives of the disable.

Birth defect is increasing on a large scale due to the use of radioactive materials and gas warfare. The transformation of a radioactive substance into highly lethal airborne aerosol is examined to be a dangerous weapon of mass destruction. The use of depleted uranium (DU) during the war between Israel and Egypt back in October 1973 clearly shows how dangerous the continued use of such chemical weapon can be.

Childbearing is to become a punishable crime. Population control advocates believe that if the desired balance between the earth and its human population could not be restored through some intelligent and rational means, such as industrialization, brutal environmentalists may deploy more radical means which is totally anti-human. Means such as contamination of food and water supply, mercury tainting of staple foods, pesticides and cloned meat are dangerous to health. These are the prime cause of cancer, infertility, sterility, premature death, mental disorder, deformity, organ failure, miscarriages, and brain tumour. However, delaying pregnancy in women through vaccination will accompany a new government law that will mandate every woman to be using contraceptive chemicals, development of new vaccines that could make a woman at their childbearing age sterile.

Paul Ehrlich in his book *The Population Bomb* said:

> We have to take away from humans in the long run their reproductive autonomy as the only way to guarantee the advancement of mankind; one plan often mentioned involves the addition of temporary sterilants to water supplies or staple food. Doses of the antidote would be carefully rationed by the government to produce the desired population size.

Theodore Roosevelt also wishes that the wrong people could be entirely prevented from bleeding. Criminals should be sterilized and feeble-minded person forbidden to leave offspring behind. The emphasis should be laid on getting the desired people to breed.

The world has about 7.8 billion people. Reducing the world population by 90 per cent, according to Bill Gates, would leave the world with an estimated 500 million people. At that time, the earth would gain more structure and balance; the surviving global elites may destroy the entire industrial infrastructure and see wilderness returning throughout the world. The elites would then become responsible for the management and utilization of all the resources and amenities present on earth. Half a billion people could live a sustainable life in relative comfort. However, a large number of the public point accusing finger at the New World Order organization as the key player in executing the depopulation scheme in an attempt to achieve a one-world government.

The Illuminati pre-eminent leaders are calling for global governance. The ambition to achieve a police state with almost all government is as old as the earth. To achieve such desire requires a large-scale policy of population control and the cooperation of every human entity to participate in the adventure of population reduction. The concept of globalization outlines the process by which regional economies, societies, and cultures have become integrated through a global network of political ideas, communication transportation, and trade.

The outcome of global transformation will cause all men to accept the New World Order. The Illuminati godfathers and the world decision-makers will create a new world of smart species, a new society where intelligent people evolve around every community. It will be a society of only the super-rich, a stress-free world made of more mature beings. Having a number of people on earth under control is one of the best ways proposed to achieve a one-world government, and population control remains the responsibility of every government. The economic implication of high population growth in the Third World is severe. The advocates believe that at the success of complete elimination of the unwanted people on earth, the planetary regime would be left with less people to do ecological damage.

The global depopulation technologies and instrument have been under development for decades. It is no longer a hidden agenda to a lot of people in the public that many of these man-made disasters which involve mass extermination, such as the Jewish Holocaust during the dark days of World War II, are part of depopulation plot. The flu pandemic, which killed an estimated 20 million people worldwide between 1918 and 1919, clearly identifies the effectiveness of the depopulation scheme at its infancy. The same movement that led to the massacre of Christians in Rwanda by Hutu forces in June 1994 has grown stronger and unstoppable in recent times. In that incident, thousands of defenceless Christians were murdered while other tens of thousands were mercilessly killed in hospitals and schools. Many opinions refer this as a dirty event aimed to trigger civil war in order to achieve mass destruction.

The population control advocates argue that war and birth control seem not the quickest means to curtail population growth. Other active devices, such as bacteriological war, could possibly be employed so as to achieve fast results. An advanced form of biological warfare that targets a specific genotype has become a useful political instrument.

Many populists had demonstrated that in order to re-establish the balance in population growths, the government has to introduce compulsory population control laws. A law that covers compulsory abortion should be sustained in the existing constitution; reproductive health-care services will then become the government's primary function. Abortion in some way has proven to fit the bill. It is estimated that over 1 billion lives have been terminated through abortion programme sponsored by the government of a highly industrialized nation. In many nations, a pregnant schoolchild is forcibly taken to abortion clinic without the parents' notification. The hidden secret behind the sudden decline in lifespan of Russian men is troubling; the average lifespan of a Russian male had fallen from 68 years in 1985 to 57.7 years in 1994. The Chinese revolution and the social experiment in China under Chairman Mao's leadership and the rolling out one-child policy marked great achievement.

The deep meaning of the message found on the Georgia Guidestones, which in other words can be translated as the New World Order commandments, interconnected with the New Earth Rule on planetary conservation, reads:

> Maintain humanity under 500,000,000 in perpetual balance with nature.
>
> Guide reproduction wisely, improving fitness and diversity.
>
> Unite humanity with a living new language.
>
> Rule passion-faith-tradition and all things with tempered reason.
>
> Protect people and nations with fair laws and just courts.
>
> Let all nations rule internally, resolving external disputes in a World Court.
>
> Avoid petty laws and useless officials.
>
> Balance personal rights with social duties.
>
> Price truth-beauty-love-seeking harmony with the infinite.

Be not a cancer on the earth.

Leave room for nature.

Leave room for nature.

The above message was inscribed in eight different languages on the four great pillars of the American Stonehenge, and it is directly related to the future of humanity. According to population advocates, this new scientific religion will demand its holocaust a sacred victim; by means of drug and injection, the population will induce to accept whatever choice his scientific masters has chosen.

The implementation of a New World Order policy is no longer a hidden agenda. All initiatives, programmes, and plans were written out for the public view. The elites believe that by letting the public understand the master plan, some may support their mission while others would better get prepared against the inevitable consequences.

Other radical means proposed to combat population growth may involve mass starvation, covert neo-engineering, and genetically modified food. Depression, drugs, and addiction were agents of mind control and the root cause of suicide. It is estimated that over 1 million people die by suicide worldwide annually; that represents 16 deaths per 10,000 populations. An average of one person dies by suicide every forty seconds somewhere in the world.

The Illuminati are using pornography as a primary mind slavery tool to gain access into the mind file of millions of people. Lucifer has poured the spirit of lust upon the surface of the earth, deteriorating the emotional value of the weak-minded and leaving the victims with loss of personality.

One might want to ask why gay rights movements have increased over the past ten years. The number of same-sex marriage is spiralling out of control. Netherland became the first country to legalize same-sex marriage in the world, and about nine other countries have passed gay rights into the bill.

Sex education is encouraged all over the world, and free distribution of condom has multiple sponsors across the globe. The theme of all these works is to control population growth. Population reduction is one must-achieve plan of the ruling class. The big players in the game want all the minorities to be eliminated so that the earth will become sustainable for them to occupy. According to Zbigniew Brzezinski, 'The capacity to impose control over humanity is at historically low. It is easier to kill a million people rather than trying to control a million people.'

We are living in an era of accelerated knowledge. The ambition of the elite will drag the human race to a breaking point. The age of human transformation is the age when all the vices of mankind will culminate and wage war against humanity. The elites and the super-rich are worried too. They are scared of the future of humanity. The think tank knows that the human race will not survive; they have envisioned the doomsday and have imagined the horrible nature of human future, so they are planning a way of escape.

'The world's super-rich people are prepared for the consequences of man's inhumanity to man. Some are buying airstrips while others are buying underground bunkers. Some may run to hide in another planet, leaving the helpless poor to bear the agony of the 'final earth disaster'. Scientists, doctors, and entrepreneurs are willing to pay high to secure ultra-modern building that will be resistance to nuclear attack. The elites know that social inequality will trigger more civil unrest, and there will be total violence across every nation. Nemesis will catch up with the earth.

In the wake of the uncontrollable economic crisis, famine will usher in with full force. The gap between the rich and the poor will become unimaginable. There shall be an increase in crime in an attempt to survive, especially among the youth. There shall be sharp divisible in the activities of man. The rich will tend to oppress the poor. Slavery shall slowly return in a very modern way. There shall be recreation of new laws that protect only the rich. The poor will remain insecure.

Global governance cannot tolerate individual freedom or rights to private property. Education and enlightenment will rightfully belong to the wealthy families. The poor will be denied education. The rich may destroy the poor through super-intelligent means. The journey of a human being on earth is far beyond our collective imagination. We find ourselves in a situation which we did not choose nor have the capacity to alter. It is necessary for everyone to embrace education. One needs knowledge to be protected and secured in this world of wars. Prepare your children's future with sound education as you do not know what may likely be the next challenge. Knowledge keeps you informed and updates you in every stage of your life. Knowledge makes you appreciate yourself even when some people might consider you unimportant.

Education should be a priority for everyone. The elites could not allow all human to acquire a high level of education and enlightenment because when every human would acquired sufficient knowledge, there could be nowhere the elites could hide for their crimes against humanity.

The selfish nature of a man will cause him to reflect when it is too late to turn back the hands of time.

Chapter

10 Message of Truth

Good people, today I bring to you a message of truth and enlightenment, a universal truth with no substitute. Our journey so far in this world is indeed marked by catastrophe and tragedies. The future of our happiness is largely determined by our total declaration and acceptance of the truth as the fundamental footprint in achieving a happy state of living which we ever long for. To introduce a new society that is free of the pains and agony, we must be open to the truth and be willing to fight, persuade, and conquer any fears that may arise against the truth that we seek.We must understand that we are in a race and must be prepared and be vigilant.

Our destiny has designed us to run a race in which our success cannot be predicted by mere looking at our physical fitness and emotional strength; rather, our success in this journey will be determined by the capacity of our spiritual well-being and our zeal to embrace the truth and accept what is morally right. Our quest to discover the truth and find comfort in life did not actually kick off in our present day. It has been running for ages by those that existed before our time. We have seen the limitation and weakness of the first runners (the previous generation). We are privileged to take advantage of the failure of the old generation to conquer every challenge that may attack the truth that we seek in our today's world.

This race can be troublesome and life-threatening at the expense of our confidence and free will to live. We must all buckle up and tighten up our shoelaces. The track line of this race is guided by a sharp metal so that anyone who slips on this single track line pierces his toes, so we must race with caution.

Right from creation, the human race has been characterized with pains and misery from the time he violated the rules of the garden and has totally lost the chance of living a fulfilled and promising life. In our modern world, our immediate desire is to live beyond all limitations. Everyone wants to live a stress-free life full of abundance and provision from nature in a new world of peace where pure love unites everyone together as one family—a brave new world where racism, culture, language, colour and religious sceptics have lost their power to create war and terrorism.

We must rise up against our weakness and be responsible for our change. The historical account of human existence has shown a man's inability to uphold his destiny. The effort required to protect and secure the dignity of a human person is also our single or collective responsibility, but trying to lay blame on our peripheral circumstances is baseless as nothing could be held accountable for our failure and shortcoming; therefore, we must strive to live beyond all obstacles. The threats and challenges we face today are greatly influenced by our mental capacity.

The limitation in our thinking ability and objection towards learning still keep us in the dark, and we keep on wandering like a sheep without a shepherd. That is to say that we have completely lost our way. Education is light, and ignorance is darkness. To seek knowledge is a sacred duty. In Islam, the first word revealed of the holy Quran was 'Iqra', which can be translated into 'read' or 'learn'. Acquire education and live happily ever after.

Whoever follows a path in pursuit of knowledge, God will make a path to paradise easy for him. Knowledge is light, and ignorance is a shame. Knowledge brings a great reward and brings balance to life. Knowledge removes the darkness of ignorance in life and makes you joyful. Without knowledge, we remain depressed in life. Knowledge makes you feel better and appreciate yourself. It offers great protection and guards you against insecurity. Continuous learning makes one feel accomplished and also equips you with words to say to others.

Knowledge helps one to make the right decision in order to avoid depression. Knowledge interconnects with wisdom, and therein, we find plane road to success. To acquire proper knowledge of the nature and its surrounding is the surest way to relate to our environment, thereby exercising dominance over all activities of life and bringing every other factor under human control. Knowledge is confidence. Knowledge is power.

The world is designed with beauty and smile, so what is the essence of crying? We have everything to live on, lots to hold on to, and much more to refresh upon. Comparing perspective of death to human survival, it is obvious that we are enjoying the privilege of temporal existence here on earth. Sooner or later, our souls will be separated from our bodies, and this incident will automatically usher us into another realm of life that is quite unclear to a mere mortal. Every soul will be subjected to death; nothing will remain static here. Our bodies, our homes, our professions, our possessions, our values, our personalities, our dignity, our prestige, and our ambition will all be wiped away someday. So why are we spending our *calculated time* fighting and hating one another? What is the need for killing when all flesh will be subjected to death?

To the government and the leaders, to the powerful rulers and those who exercise the veto power, to those who make laws and those who execute the law, to the governing body and those who are governed, it's time to wake up and claim what is rightfully ours. Freedom, good health, happiness, peace, comfort, sound education, and personal development are our primary rights, and nothing could stop us from living like a normal person while enjoying the free gifts of nature. This is the time to sit up and live above corruption and injustice. The leaders must have a grain of compassion in their hearts in order to feel the pain and agony their followers are going through due to unfair leadership and ill treatment.

In some part of the world, people are living in executive mansions. They have access to the luxurious amenities of life. Their world is at their fingertips. They are ruling their world, and they wish they never experience death. On the other part of the world, people are living in slums. Many are dying of starvation. Some do not have access to drinking water; thus, their life expectancy is very short. There is little or no employment opportunity, and this gives rise to organized crimes, fraud, armed robberies, terrorism, child abuse, human trafficking, street hawking, bribery, and all sorts of social vices—all in an attempt to survive.

Some could no longer bear the pain that life has inflicted on them, and they have chosen to take away their own lives, thinking that death is the absolute solution. But remember, we are all one people created by one Supreme Being. This is the right time to stand firm against social vices. Each country in the world is challenged with a unique problem, but we must come to terms with one another and pursue our common goal. The root cause of our predicament is insincerity to one's own self. We must be guided by a common truth in order to eliminate man's inhumanity to man. We must show love and compassion to one another and must not be misled by superstition. We have to remove impurity inside our minds and adjust the way we think about others. Pride and arrogance kill a man a hundred times before his death. We must do away with the mentality of the ruling class— the presidents and the prime ministers, the bankers, and the royal family. We should understand that we are one people with common aspirations, and we are going through common struggle in life, so we need to show love.

The future of our species is solely in our hands and has become our respective obligation. When we finally define the form of life which we intend for our forthcoming generation, then we shall aim to maintain a sustainable development. In order to achieve this vision, we must be willing to build a developed society with highly educated people that will stimulate the transformation that we seek. It is extremely necessary to eradicate ignorance. In many villages, people do not have the finance to send their children to school. The kids do not study, and they keep on living and suffering on the dark side of life. Learned people are becoming scarce in the backward regions. Most of these people were forgotten by the government. No one cares for them. They live like outcasts in the zone where they rightfully belong. Non-government organizations are doing their best by extending charity, but more effort is needed from the government.

Science and technology has a way of improving life very fast. We need to embrace and welcome advancements in science. The development of technology has obviously slowed in the developing countries and many other emerging economies. These nations are dependent on the technological achievements of highly industrialized nations. Information is said to be the quickest means to induce economic and social development, but until the twenty-first century, African nations had failed to produce a well-functioning and advanced information technology. As of 2013, African countries account for only 16 per cent of the world's Internet users. This figure is very poor when compared to 61 per cent and 75 per cent of the Internet users in America and Europe respectively. More projects and budgets should be designed by the government, focusing on technological advancement. There is also the need to offer the youths access to practical science rather than theory so that their knowledge shall not be limited to the introduction to technology. Building and promoting talents as well as setting up a solid medical research teams is advisable.

It is also important to take a critical look at the negative impact of overpopulation on climate change. The effect of overpopulation on emerging economies is hazardous due to insufficient supply of resources needed to fuel up economic growth in order to achieve a sustainable development. In order to control excessive population, a source of clean method has to be applied. Adoption of effective family planning policy and childbirth regulation is an efficient way to achieve this goal.

Ebola disaster will hit badly on the economic growth of the countries in West Africa, according to a recent report released by UN Development Programme, which states that 'West Africa as a whole may lose an average of at least 3.6 billion dollar per year between 2014 to 2017, due to a decrease in trade, closing of borders, flight cancellations and reduced Foreign Direct Investment and tourist activity, fuelled by stigma'. But notwithstanding the challenges and difficulties this incident imposed on our nations, we shall continue to struggle to overcome the battle. We shall defeat Ebola virus and its consequences, and then Ebola will become part of our history. We shall sit back and enjoy the peace and unity that we ever hope for. We shall hold hands together with one another, travel to any country of our choice without restriction or fear of isolation. Our life will totally come back to normal.

Finally, we must remember the promises we made to our Mother Nation and the covenant we had with our forefathers, who worked hard and sacrificed their lives for our freedom. We have a pledge to a dear nation to be faithful, loyal, and honest, to serve our nation with all our strength, to defend her unity and uphold her honour and glory, so help us God.

Powered By

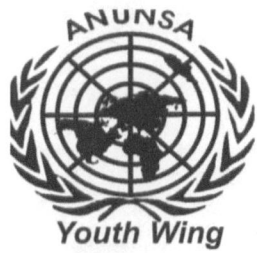

Youth Wing

All Nigerian United Nations' Students & Youth Association

For enquiries:

Email: *ebola_info@dr.com*

Tel: *+2348107257036*

Lighting Source UK Ltd.
Milton Keynes UK
UKOW04F0142300915

9 7814 8 2807691